The H.O.P.E. Formula:
The Ultimate Health Secret

By Brenda Watson, N.D.

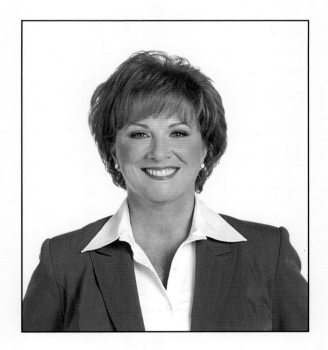

with Suzin Stockton, M.A.
Foreword by Leonard Smith, M.D.

The H.O.P.E. Formula: The Ultimate Health Secret

By Brenda Watson, N.D., C.T.
with Suzin Stockton, M.A.
Foreword by Leonard Smith, M.D.

ISBN 0-9719309-4-5

First Printing
Renew Life Press and Information Services
2076 Sunnydale Drive
Clearwater, FL 33765
1-866-450-1784

Acknowledgements

The gratitude and thanks I feel for all the teachers in my life goes beyond the list here. The thousands of clients with whom I have worked and the people to whom I've lectured across the country were the inspiration to create this book. The need for simplification of the digestion and detoxification processes is the primary motivation for this book.

I thank Suzin Stockton for her help and guidance in creating this book. Her persistence in keeping me focused on this project is the reason we have this finished book. Her vast knowledge of natural healing and writing contributed greatly to the shaping of this book.

Thank you, Leonard Smith M.D., for your contribution of information and unique perspectives, traditional as well as holistic. Also, your constant optimism and love helped make this an easier process.

To the family of ReNew Life and Advanced Naturals, your love and constant support of me and the endeavors of the company make me very grateful and proud. I could not have asked for a better support group during this process. A special thanks to Kathi Murray for her knowledge and creativity in the design of this book.

A special thanks to my children (Joy and Travis) who have been instrumental in this process of creating a support system for me.

Most of all, I wish to acknowledge my husband, Stan Watson, for his constant support and participation in the writing and editing of this book. His endless support has been one of the main reasons for my success in this field. He has been unselfish in creating the space for me to travel endlessly with this message.

Brenda Watson, N.D., C.T.
Clearwater, FL
2006

Preface

After many years of lecturing across the country to thousands of people about the digestive system and the detoxification process, I began to think about writing this book. At each lecture I knew the explanation of the digestive process needed to be simplified and made "real" to people through the use of pictures and charts. Such visual aids make the information easier to understand.

My personal struggle with poor health made me aware that digestive health is important, whether you're trying to regain health (as I was) or maintain it. In either case, detoxifying the body (ridding it of poisons) and improving the digestive process are necessary.

I regained my health many years ago largely through colon hydrotherapy and herbal supplementation. At that time, such therapeutic practices as fasting and colonics were considered "strange" by most people. The natural healing philosophy has become more accepted during the last two decades, and so too have such therapies. The holistic approach to healing is being increasingly viewed as "scientific" with the accreditation of a growing number of naturopathic colleges. The development and use of specialized laboratory tests to aid physicians in diagnosing such digestive disorders as dysbiosis has also made natural healing philosophy and practices more acceptable.

During my career, I have worked in – and developed my own – clinics that specialize in digestion and detoxification. In doing so, I have seen many people regain their health and better maintain it through the application of natural healing principles. This has inspired me and given rise to a passion for my work – a passion that remains to this day, which has resulted in a renewed commitment to health education.

I am confident that the information contained in this book will enable you, the reader, to better understand the digestive system and its function. Knowledge is power. The information in *The H.O.P.E. Formula: The Ultimate Health Secret* will empower you to make the best health choices and quite literally renew your life! It has been said that "the digestive system is like the roots of a tree; when the roots are diseased, the whole tree is affected." Nutrition, digestion, absorption, bacterial balance and intestinal permeability all play interdependent functions in the health of the gastrointestinal tract and the health of the whole body. All are presented in this book.

Brenda Watson, N.D., C.T.

P.S. In reading through this book, you'll note that at times I use the word "I," and at other times, I use the word "we." "I" is used when the opinion expressed or experience described is my own. When "we" is used, that opinion/experience is one that is shared by my co-author, Suzin Stockton.

Foreword

As a board-certified surgeon, I have, during the last 25 years, operated on thousands of people with digestive disorders. By the time these patients arrive at my office they are often well into a chronic disease state. I have often asked myself, "What could this person have done to avoid this surgery?" In many cases, the answer is that these operations could have been prevented with diet and lifestyle modifications. Going a step further, I am convinced that the majority of all diseases could be avoided or modified with a proper understanding of nutrition, digestion, elimination and stress modification.

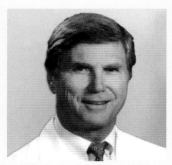

These "digestive care" concepts are not new: Taking the time to eat clean food, chewing thoroughly, eating probiotics (good bacteria like acidophilus and bifidobacteria), taking digestive enzymes, eating raw foods, and consuming optimum amounts of fiber and essential fatty acids are basic health guidelines that have been known and practiced worldwide for thousands of years. Our modern society has diluted these key digestive concepts with advertisements for "fast food," fad diets and medical advice that promotes a variety of pills in an attempt to control digestive problems rather than address the causes. Proper digestion, elimination and detoxification are the cornerstones of vibrant health. The skyrocketing incidence of chronic illnesses in the U.S.A. will continue until we embrace and promote these digestive care concepts.

The medical literature is replete with clinical data to support the various facets of digestive care and detoxification. Many of the books on the subject are as difficult to read as the clinical studies. Brenda Watson has done an excellent job defining and clarifying the most important digestive care principles. This book is complete in its attention to data but simple in the delivery of the information. Both medical practitioners and all others interested in digestive care and detoxification will find this book to be most helpful in increasing their understanding in this area.

Leonard Smith, M.D.
Gainesville, Florida, 2006

Table of Contents

Healthy Digestive System

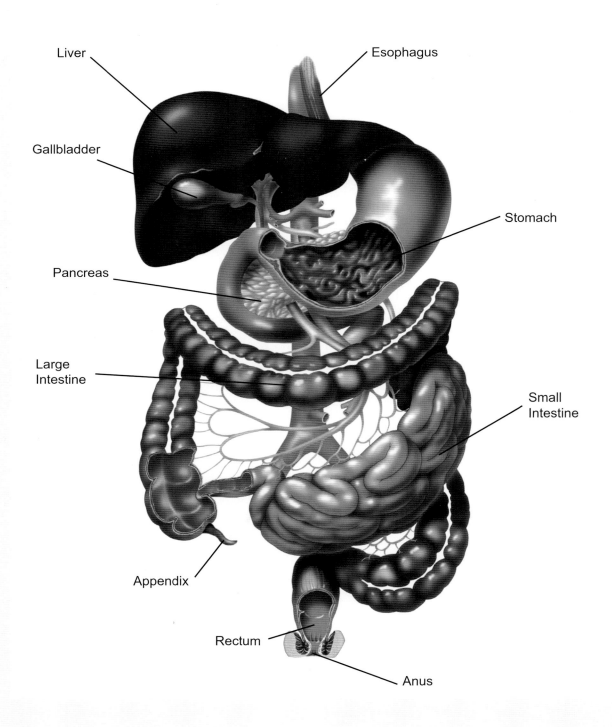

Liver

Esophagus

Gallbladder

Stomach

Pancreas

Large Intestine

Small Intestine

Appendix

Rectum

Anus

Unhealthy Digestive System

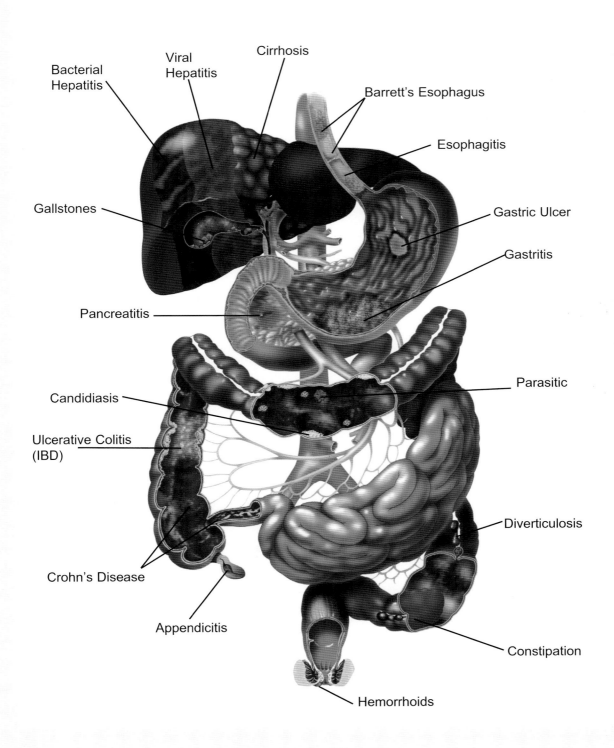

Bacterial Hepatitis

Viral Hepatitis

Cirrhosis

Barrett's Esophagus

Esophagitis

Gallstones

Gastric Ulcer

Gastritis

Pancreatitis

Candidiasis

Parasitic

Ulcerative Colitis (IBD)

Crohn's Disease

Diverticulosis

Appendicitis

Constipation

Hemorrhoids

Introduction

What is more valuable to you than good health? Your family? Your faith in a higher power? A hefty bank balance? A good movie? A new car? Well, guess what? You can't enjoy any of them if you have poor health. If you are sick, exhausted, or in pain, you will simply not have the time or energy to enjoy all the things that life has to offer. You will spend all your time, money and energy trying to deal with your poor health, rather than creating a better life for yourself, your family, your community and maybe even the rest of us.

"So," you may ask, "what can I do about my poor health?" Well, you can do a great deal. With very few exceptions, we do not suddenly wake up one day with poor health. I'll let you in on a secret: We create our own poor health. How do we do that? Well, we eat too much, drink too much, exercise too little and generally abuse our bodies over a long period of time. We live stressful lives in stressful cities that are full of too many people. We breathe toxic air, drink polluted water and generally pass bacteria and viruses around so often that it is amazing we survive at all. The fact that we do survive for decades in relatively good health is, in part, a testament to the strength of our digestive systems. That's right, I said "our digestive systems." It is not natural to drink chlorinated water or homogenized milk; nor are we naturally designed to eat food that has been irradiated, filled with preservatives or coated with pesticides, but that's what we do every day. Through it all, our digestive systems function for years to break down foods and liquids into the few nutrients that are available. Our digestive systems don't stop there. They also help to filter and eliminate toxins, parasites, fungi, bacteria and viruses. It has long been known that health comes from the body's ability to digest nutrients and

eliminate waste. The digestive system is responsible for assuring that you:

• Digest foods completely
• Eliminate wastes naturally

The more efficiently your body performs these functions, the healthier you are likely to be.

Do you remember the saying, "You are what you eat?" There is certainly truth in it. More accurately however, you are what you digest (break down), absorb (take into the bloodstream) and assimilate (take into the cells). The problem is that not all the food we consume is properly utilized. Even assuming that we eat the highest quality food available (most of us do not), we cannot achieve optimal health unless our digestive systems are functioning at their peak.

Aging, poor food quality, faulty preparation methods, external toxins or parasites can lead to a premature decline of our digestive systems and long-term chronic disease. These diseases can include arthritis, diabetes, fibromyalgia, chronic fatigue, Alzheimer's, irritable bowel syndrome and many others. When our digestive systems do not function correctly, we are not able to reap the full benefit of the food we eat, regardless of how nutrient-dense it may be. Proper digestion is only half the story: To achieve optimal health, our bodies or systems must also eliminate wastes and toxins quickly and efficiently.

Proper elimination of toxins is particularly problematic. In today's world, more than ever, we are exposed to a wide variety of toxins: They're in our air, food and water, in the workplace and at home. We even generate toxins within our own bodies. These toxins produce irritation and inflammation, adding to the burden of the digestive system. When the digestive system becomes overwhelmed, it is no longer able to adequately perform detoxification functions. This is a condition called "toxic overload."

Now, before you quit your stressful job, obtain a divorce, move to the forest and live in a cave, you may want to think about what you can do to keep your digestive system healthy. Unfortunately, you can't do much about your age, but you can help your digestive system function at optimal levels by giving your body the proper nutrients and by keeping the digestive system clean and well maintained. By following the suggestions in this book, particularily the H.O.P.E. formula, you will be on your way to better health. While they are not as well known as vitamins and minerals, the H.O.P.E. elements are every bit as vital to your health and well being. The H.O.P.E. formula provides essential nourishment to your body, helping you improve your digestion, which will have the net effect of preventing disease and assisting in the restoration of health.

In the pages that follow, you will learn what happens to your food from the time it enters the mouth until it leaves the body. Furthermore, you will learn what can go wrong in the process and why. AND—most importantly—you'll learn how to avoid, as well as correct and reverse, problems with digestion and elimination. This book will provide you with the knowledge and information you need to achieve optimal and vibrant health; but as in all things in life, you must take the first step.

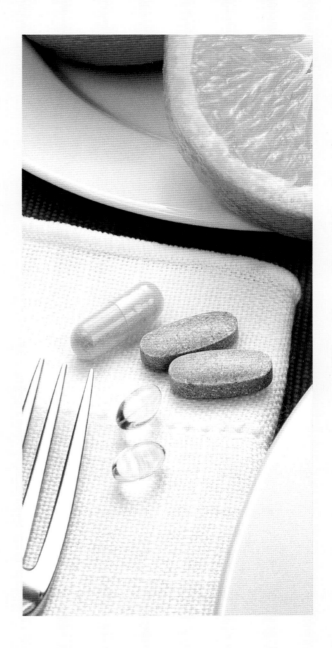

CHAPTER 1

THE HEALTHY
digestive SYSTEM

It is not what you do once in a while, but what you do everyday that greatly determines your health.

Source:
Brenda Watson, N.D., C.T.

It is estimated that as much as 40% of the population suffer from some form of digestive stress. If you are reading this book, you probably are within this group. You may be unconcerned with the details of the digestive process or just want to know how to be or become healthy. If that is your goal, then the journey to achieving that goal begins with a clear understanding of a healthy digestive system.

WHAT IS DIGESTION?

Digestion encompasses the chemical and motor (physical motion) activities that separate food into its most basic components so that they can be absorbed through the lining of the small intestine. Digestion is the process of converting food into chemical substances that can be absorbed and assimilated. It begins in the mouth and ends in the **large intestine** or **colon**.

What Does the Digestive System Do?
The digestive system has two broad functions: The first and best known is the digestion and absorption of food. The second function is the excretion of wastes. Both of these occur primarily in the small and large intestines; hence the phrase by Gloria Gilbère, N.D. (Naturopathic Doctor), "The road to health is paved with good intestines."

What Organs Make Up the Digestive System?
The digestive tract is a tube (about 30 feet long) that begins with the mouth and ends with the anus. The digestive system (or gastrointestinal tract) is made up of the mouth, esophagus, stomach, small intestine, large intestine and anus. Along this tube are accessory organs like the teeth, tongue, salivary glands, gallbladder, liver and pancreas.

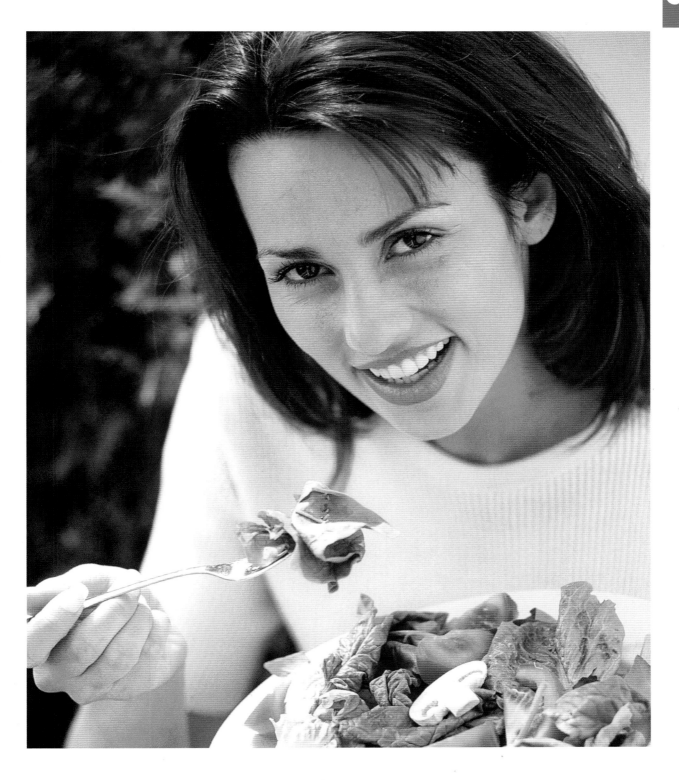

What Are the Functions of the Digestive System?

The digestive tract has three primary functions:

- **Motor** – assisting food movement
- **Secretory** – preparing food for absorption by producing digestive enzymes
- **Absorptive** – breaking food down and converting it into substances that can be absorbed through digestion

THE DIGESTIVE PROCESS

Digestion begins in the mouth where the teeth chew food into smaller particles. Then saliva coats and softens those food particles with **enzymes** (**ptyalin** and **amylase**) that break down carbohydrates (starches and sugars). Saliva also contains enzymes, such as **lysozyme**, that attack bacteria and their protein coats directly. This is the body's first line of defense against parasites and foreign invaders. Once chewing is completed (and sometimes even when it is not), food is swallowed and transferred down the **esophagus** to the stomach.

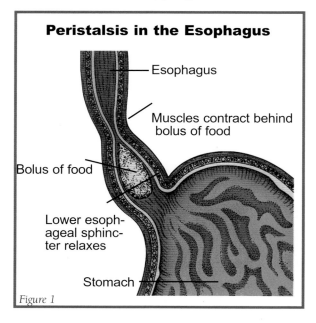

Peristalsis in the Esophagus

— Esophagus

Muscles contract behind bolus of food

Bolus of food

Lower esophageal sphincter relaxes

Stomach

Figure 1

The Esophagus

The esophagus is a 10-inch long muscular tube, lined with mucus-producing cells, which lubricates the food so that it passes through with ease. The esophagus transports food to the stomach through the action of its wave-like muscular contractions (**peristalsis**). It is coated with a protective mucous lining. The muscular valve at the bottom of the esophagus is known as the **lower esophageal sphincter**. This valve remains tightly closed when food is not being eaten so that stomach acid cannot back into the esophagus and cause heartburn. It opens and closes quickly to allow food to pass into the **stomach**.

The Stomach

Many people are surprised to find that very little absorption actually occurs in the stomach. The mucous cells of the stomach can absorb some water, short-chain fatty acids and certain drugs, such as alcohol and aspirin, but the stomach is essentially a holding and mixing tank for food. Its main functions are storage and preliminary digestion. The stomach functions like a big blender, churning and liquefying food. The properly functioning stomach secretes five

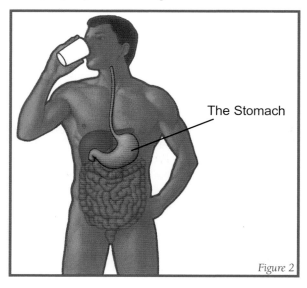

The Stomach

Figure 2

important substances: (1) mucus, (2) **hydrochloric acid** (HCl), (3) a precursor of the protein-digesting enzyme **pepsin**, (4) **gastrin**, a hormone to regulate acid production and (5) gastric **lipase**, which assists in the digestion of fat.

A mucous lining coats the cells of the stomach to protect them from the HCl and enzymes that must be present for proper digestion. This alkaline mucous lining can be damaged by dehydration, over-consumption of food or aspirin, or by the bacterium **Helicobacter pylori** (H. pylori). This damage can often lead to **gastritis** (irritation of the stomach lining) or to a stomach ulcer.

> Contrary to popular belief, many Americans who suffer from heartburn produce too little hydrocloric acid (HCl), not too much. Without enough HCl, you may not be able to sufficiently break down proteins. This can lead to bloating, gas and heartburn. Low HCl production can also result in problems with bacterial infections or parasites.

Hydrochloric acid (HCl) is produced by **parietal** cells (tiny pumps) in the lining of the stomach. This acid is needed to ensure the proper functioning of the stomach. HCl has two primary functions: It provides the acidic environment necessary for the enzyme pepsin to break down proteins; and it helps prevent infection by destroying most parasites and bacteria.

At the end of the stomach is the **pyloric sphincter**, which controls the opening between the end of the stomach and the **duodenum**, the first section of the small intestine.

The Duodenum

When food leaves the stomach, it enters the first section of the small intestine known as the duodenum. It is now called chyme, a mixture of food, HCl and mucus, which is approximately the consistency of split pea soup. As the duodenum fills, hormones released from the duodenal lining (1) delay gastric emptying, (2) promote bile flow from the liver and gallbladder and (3) promote secretion of water, bicarbonate and potent digestive enzymes from the pancreas. The surface of the duodenum is smooth for the first few inches, but quickly changes to a surface with many folds and small finger-like projections called villi or microvilli (very small projections). These projections serve to increase the surface area and absorption capabilities of the duodenum. Properly functioning accessory organs (liver, gallbladder and pancreas) are crucial during this first stage of digestion.

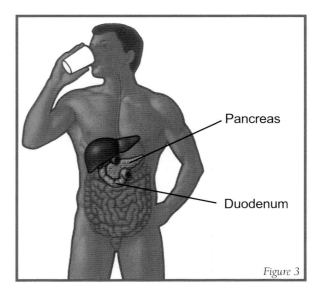

Pancreas

Duodenum

Figure 3

The Pancreas

The **pancreas** is a 6-inch long accessory organ that has three main functions important to digestion:

1. Neutralizes stomach acid
2. Regulates blood sugar levels
3. Produces digestive enzymes

Digestive enzymes digest proteins, carbohydrates and fats. The **proteolytic** (protein-digesting pancreatic) enzymes are secreted in an inactive form and are only activated once they reach the duodenum. The other pancreatic enzymes are secreted in an active form but require **ions** (electrically charged molecules) or bile to be present for optimal activity. Bicarbonates are alkaline and serve to neutralize stomach acid and activate digestive enzymes. These secretions (pancreatic enzymes and bicarbonates) are delivered directly into the duodenum, the upper portion of the small intestine. The pancreas also secretes hormones which help manage blood sugar levels, directly into the bloodstream. These hormones are **insulin** (sugar lowering) and **glucagon** (sugar raising).

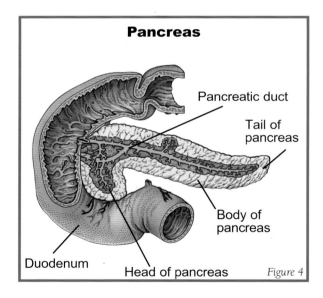

Pancreas

Pancreatic duct

Tail of pancreas

Body of pancreas

Duodenum

Head of pancreas

Figure 4

The Liver and Gallbladder

The **liver** has several important functions, a number of which are related to digestion. It produces approximately 85% of the body's **cholesterol** (only about 15% comes from food). About 80% of the cholesterol produced by the liver is used to make **bile**. Bile is composed of bile salts, hormones (including cholesterol) and toxins. It acts to emulsify and distribute fat, cholesterol and

---

The Pancreas Produces

Bicarbonate – neutralizes stomach acid

Enzymes – digest carbohydrates, fats and protein

Insulin – regulates blood sugar levels

---

fat-soluble vitamins throughout the intestines. Bile is an alkaline substance that neutralizes stomach acid. Between meals, it is stored in the gallbladder, a pear-shaped organ located just below the liver. When food (chyme) enters the duodenum, a signal is sent to the gallbladder to contract, thereby releasing bile into the **small intestine**.

The Small Intestine

Ninety percent of all nutrients are absorbed in the small intestine, the body's major digestive organ. The small intestine resembles a coiled hose and is approximately 20-25 feet long. It is here that most food is completely digested and absorbed. The small intestine contains cells that serve many functions: Some produce mucus, some make enzymes, some absorb nutrients and others are capable of killing bacteria. The cells are arranged in folds upon folds, which force the chyme to move slower so it can be broken down completely and absorbed. These folds also increase the surface area of the **mucosa**, the thin mucous membrane lining the walls of the small intestine.

The small intestine consists of three sections—the **duodenum**, the **jejunum** and the **ileum**. The duodenum (first foot of the small intestine) connects to the jejunum, which in turn connects to the ileum. The duodenum primarily absorbs minerals. The jejunum absorbs water-soluble vitamins, carbohydrates and proteins. The ileum absorbs fat-soluble vitamins, fat, cholesterol and bile salts. The walls of the small intestine secrete alkaline digestive enzymes, which continue the separation of foods—proteins into amino acids, fats into fatty acids and glycerin and carbohydrates into simple sugars.

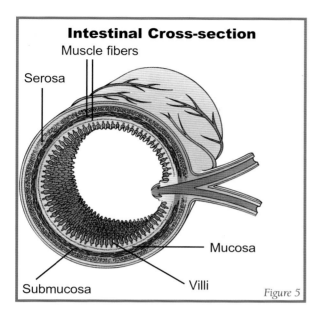

Intestinal Cross-section

Muscle fibers

Serosa

Mucosa

Submucosa

Villi

Figure 5

The Colon or Large Intestine

The last organ through which food residue passes is the colon or large intestine. The three major segments are the **ascending** (right side of body), **transverse** (connects right to left side) and **descending** (left side). Chyme enters the ascending colon through the **ileocecal valve** (ICV), a one-way valve that connects the small and large intestines and regulates the flow of chyme entering the large intestine. The ICV is designed to let waste pass into the colon and prevent it from backing into the small intestine. When chyme passes through the ICV, and then into the very lowest portion of the ascending colon, known as the **cecum**, it is still in a liquid state. The cecum is the first section of the five feet of colon. Food waste travels up the ascending colon (through rhythmic waves of contraction or peristalsis), across the transverse and down the descending portion of the organ. As it moves across the transverse colon, liquid is extracted. It is the job of the colon to absorb water and nutrients from the chyme and to form feces. The fecal matter is in a semi-solid state, gradually becoming firmer, as it approaches the descending colon. About

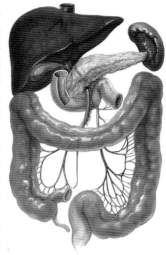

two-thirds of stool is water, undigested fiber and food products; one-third is living and dead bacteria (bacteria naturally live in the colon). The lowest portion of the descending colon is the **sigmoid**. The sigmoid colon empties into the rectum. In this area, three valves regulate the fecal matter. They are called the **valves of Houston**. This area is normally empty unless defecation is in process.

Final stages of digestion occur in the colon with the absorption of water and nutrients not absorbed by the small intestine. The liquid and nutrients are absorbed through the intestinal wall, collected by the blood vessels in the wall lining and carried to the liver through the portal vein for filtration.

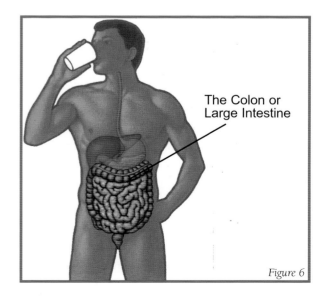

The Colon or Large Intestine

Figure 6

The large intestine also:

1. Secretes bicarbonate to neutralize acid end products
2. Stores waste products, bacteria and intestinal gas
3. Excretes poisons and waste products from the body

The **rectum** is the chamber at the end of the large intestine. Fecal matter passes into the rectum, creating the urge to defecate. The **anus** is the opening at the far end of the digestive tract. The anus allows fecal matter to pass out of the body. The anal sphincters keep the anus closed.

The Mucous Membrane

The walls of both the small and large intestines consist of four layers. The innermost layer of the small intestine is called the mucosa. The mucosa has two very important functions: First, it is designed to allow nutrients of the proper size to pass through it and into the bloodstream. Second, the mucosa blocks the passage of undigested food particles, parasites, bacteria and toxins into the bloodstream. Therefore, the mucosa or mucosal lining is a vital part of the body's immune system because it limits the volume of potential invaders. The mucosa is lined with **villi** and **microvilli**. The villi are moving absorptive cells that "suck up" small particles of digested food. On each of the villi are thousands of tiny projections of the membrane of the cell called microvilli. These little brush-like fuzzy structures (called the "**brush border**") further amplify the surface area of the small intestine. **Stretched end to end with all its folds, the small intestine has the approximate surface area of a tennis court.**

On the surface of this mucosal lining is a thick mucous layer whose surface (the **glycocalyx**) is highly viscous (slippery). Much of the mucus

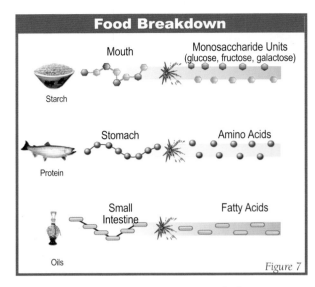

Food Breakdown

Mouth — Starch — Monosaccharide Units (glucose, fructose, galactose)

Stomach — Protein — Amino Acids

Small Intestine — Oils — Fatty Acids

Figure 7

consists of the amino sugar **N-acetyl-glucosamine** (NAG). The body makes NAG from the amino acid **L-glutamine**. L-glutamine exists in virtually all cells, and it is one of the most prevalent amino acids in the body. Humans must have L-glutamine in order to produce NAG and have a healthy mucosal lining. The mucosal lining in a healthy person sheds and then is rebuilt every three to five days. Studies have shown that individuals suffering from any inflammatory bowel disease shed this mucosal layer at a much higher rate. This may be due to an inability to convert L-glutamine into NAG.

THE DIGESTIVE ENVIRONMENT

It is difficult to fully understand the digestive system without realizing the importance of the bacteria and microbes that live in the intestinal tract. A newborn baby has essentially no digestive bacteria. Within a few hours, the bacteria and microbes begin to colonize the digestive tract. It has been observed that breast-fed babies develop a larger colony of friendly strains of **bifidobacteria** than those who are bottle-fed. Ideally, pregnant women should supplement with the friendly bacteria

Healthy Digestive Tract

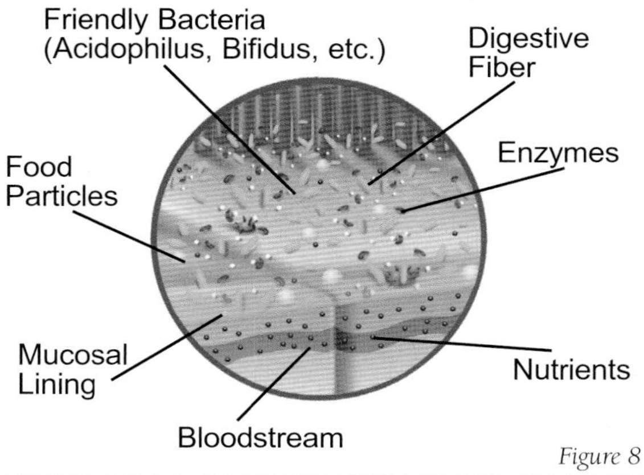

Friendly Bacteria
(Acidophilus, Bifidus, etc.)

Digestive
Fiber

Enzymes

Food
Particles

Mucosal
Lining

Nutrients

Bloodstream

Figure 8

These microbes exist throughout the digestive system from the mouth to the anus, but most of the bacteria live in the large intestine. (The stomach is so acidic that almost no bacteria can live there.) The large intestine can contain as many as four pounds of these microbial creatures at any one time. Approximately 500 different species of microbes live in the digestive system, but only 30 to 40 species constitute 99% of the microbes in the intestinal tract. In terms of how these microbes affect the body, they can be placed into one of three categories:

1. Good (or symbiotic)
2. Neutral
3. Bad

In a healthy person, there is a ratio of approximately 80–85% combined good and neutral bacteria to 15–20% bad. In many people today, this ratio is reversed. Faulty digestion can contribute to this imbalance.

The good bacteria are sometimes called "**flora**" or "**probiotics**." These good bacteria are beneficial because they:

1. Produce enzymes that help digest foods (e.g., lactase enzyme digests milk)
2. Produce the vitamins B, A and K
3. Produce **lactic acid**, which helps acidify the colon
4. Crowd bad bacteria and keep them from becoming too numerous
5. Produce organic acids that may help with fecal elimination by peristalsis
6. Produce short-chain fatty acids (**butyric acid**), which supply energy to intestinal cells

The two most important types of good bacteria are **lactobacillus** and **bifidobacteria**.

known as *Lactobacillus (L.) acidophilus*, and bifidobacteria during the third trimester of pregnancy. Friendly bacteria (also known as probiotics, discussed in chapter 6) are important for babies at the time of birth. *L. acidophilus* in the vagina inoculates the newborn as he/she passes through the birth canal, and it provides protection from other bacteria, as well as assisting with digestion and with the production of vitamins. The bifidobacteria ingested by the mother are concentrated in the breast milk and are passed on intact to the nursing baby. These two events establish the friendly bacteria in the newborn and greatly decrease the possibility of serious infections that can occur during infancy. The mother can provide friendly bacteria for her baby by ingesting a supplement containing *L. acidophilus* and bifidobacteria, or by eating yogurt or kefir with live cultures of these bacteria. It may be best to do both, since it is necessary to provide ample amounts of the probiotics on a regular basis.

> As adults, our digestive systems contain about 100 trillion bacteria, fungi and microbes. You actually have more bacteria in your gastrointestinal tract than cells in your body!

Digestive Organs

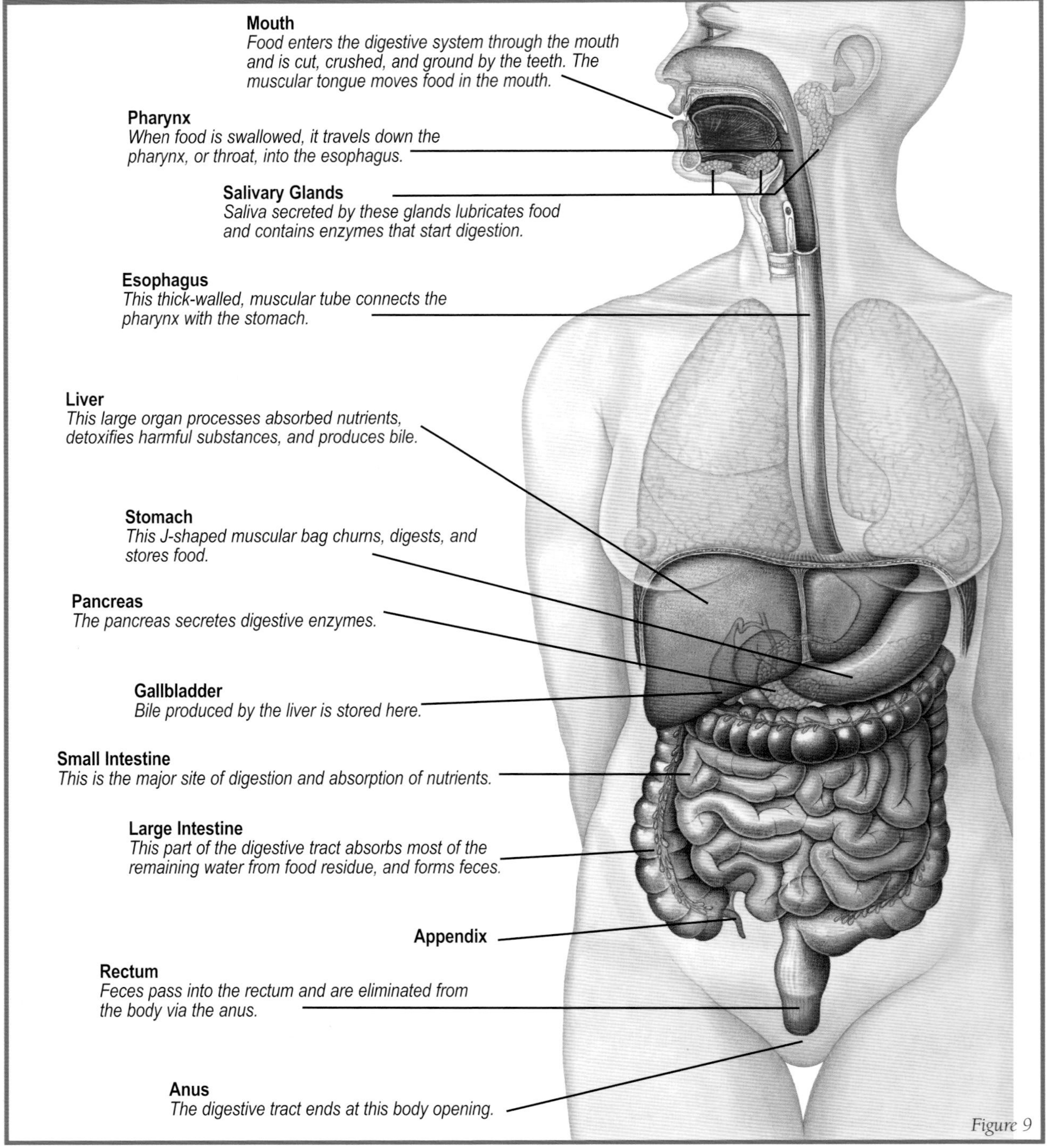

Mouth
Food enters the digestive system through the mouth and is cut, crushed, and ground by the teeth. The muscular tongue moves food in the mouth.

Pharynx
When food is swallowed, it travels down the pharynx, or throat, into the esophagus.

Salivary Glands
Saliva secreted by these glands lubricates food and contains enzymes that start digestion.

Esophagus
This thick-walled, muscular tube connects the pharynx with the stomach.

Liver
This large organ processes absorbed nutrients, detoxifies harmful substances, and produces bile.

Stomach
This J-shaped muscular bag churns, digests, and stores food.

Pancreas
The pancreas secretes digestive enzymes.

Gallbladder
Bile produced by the liver is stored here.

Small Intestine
This is the major site of digestion and absorption of nutrients.

Large Intestine
This part of the digestive tract absorbs most of the remaining water from food residue, and forms feces.

Appendix

Rectum
Feces pass into the rectum and are eliminated from the body via the anus.

Anus
The digestive tract ends at this body opening.

Figure 9

Bad bacteria produce substances that are harmful to the body. They irritate the lining of the intestines (causing gas) and can be absorbed into the bloodstream (causing disease). They cannot always be prevented from entering the body, but if the number of good and neutral bacteria stays high, then, theoretically, the bad bacteria will be kept to a minimum. Examples of bad bacteria are **salmonella** and **H. pylori**, the bacterium associated with ulcers.

The neutral bacteria are the most prevalent bacteria in the digestive tract. Neutral microbes have neither a positive nor negative impact.

The levels of these three types of organisms remain relatively constant throughout childhood and mid to late adult years. As we age, the levels of bad bacteria often increase, and the good bacteria decrease.

THE SIGNS OF GOOD DIGESTION AND ELIMINATION

At minimum, one should have one good bowel movement per day, but two to three are ideal. A "good" bowel movement is one that is walnut brown in color, with a consistency similar to toothpaste, about the length of a banana. The stool should be free of odor, leave the body easily, settle in the toilet water and gently submerge. The **transit time** for food—the elapsed time it takes for a meal to enter the mouth and then exit the rectum—should ideally be less than 24 hours. Transit time is related to exercise and the consumption of fiber and water.

> **When transit time slows, putrefied material stays in the colon longer, and toxins can enter the bloodstream through the intestinal wall.**

THE SEVEN CHANNELS OF ELIMINATION

The seven channels of elimination are:

- Colon
- Lungs
- Liver
- Skin
- Kidneys
- Blood
- Lymph

The first five of these channels (column 1) are all organs. The processes of the colon have been explained in this chapter. The liver has numerous functions and is your primary detoxification organ. The blood that flows through the vessels of the **vascular** (blood circulatory) system carries oxygen and nutrients to the cells of the body and removes harmful wastes. Not so familiar to many is the other circulatory system, the **lymphatic system**, through which **lymph** flows.

The Lymph

The **lymphatic system** and the vascular system serve to eliminate poisons from cells. The lymphatic system consists of a network of vessels that extends throughout the body, following the path of the veins. The lymphatic capillaries contain

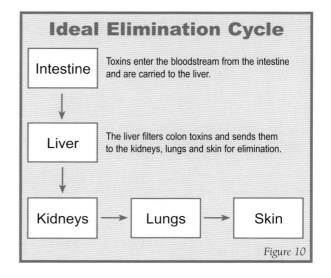

Ideal Elimination Cycle

Intestine — Toxins enter the bloodstream from the intestine and are carried to the liver.

Liver — The liver filters colon toxins and sends them to the kidneys, lungs and skin for elimination.

Kidneys → Lungs → Skin

Figure 10

a clear fluid—lymph—which carries **lympho-cytes** (immune cells). The lymphatic system is an important part of the immune system. In fact, organs of the immune system are known as "lymphoid organs." They include the following:

Bone marrow – where lymphocytes originate.

Spleen – a filter for the lymphatic system and a storage site for lymphocytes.

Liver – a major detoxification organ.

Lymph nodes – small bean-shaped structures that connect with lymphatic capillaries. (They are concentrated in the groin, armpits, neck and abdomen; they filter lymph and produce lymphocytes.)

Thymus gland – home of the **T cells**, which mobilize the body's defense system when it is immune-challenged.

All these lymphoid organs are concerned with the growth, development and deployment of white blood cells (lymphocytes), whose function it is to defend the body against **antigens** (substances the body perceives as foreign and threatening, such as viruses, fungi, bacteria, parasites and pollen).

Kidneys

The **kidneys** are two bean-shaped organs located just under the **diaphragm** in the back. The liver sends water-soluble wastes to the kidneys via the blood where this waste is eliminated through the **bladder**.

Although small enough to fit in the palm of a hand and weighing no more than an orange, the kidneys are considered the "great purifiers" of the body. Each kidney contains a million individual filter units (globules) and, according to Dr. Henry Bieler, "can filter 1700 quarts of viscous fluid

> **The gastrointestinal tract has the largest blood supply in the body, taking a third of the blood flow from the heart to get its job done.**
>
> D. Lindsey Berkson,
> *Healthy Digestion the Natural Way*

(in which 50 different chemicals are dissolved) in 24 hours."[1] The kidneys determine which of these 50 chemicals are needed by the body, absorb them and filter out the rest. Of the blood filtered by the kidneys, 0.1% becomes urine.[2] The kidneys have the additional function of maintaining water balance.

Lungs

The **lungs**, another secondary elimination organ, expel toxins from the body. One of the most common toxins is **carbon dioxide**. The action of deep breathing helps to move lymph and blood through the body, and with it, toxins. The lungs are lined with mucus and **cilia** (hair-like projections) to help protect against and remove inhaled toxins.

Skin

The **skin** is the body's largest organ. It serves as a protective barrier to prevent toxins from entering the body. Because of its size, the skin "can eliminate more cellular waste than the colon and kidneys combined."[3] It eliminates wastes through its sweat glands and mucous secretions and is considered a secondary elimination organ. The skin protects our inner parts and gauges temperature needs. New skin is made every 24 hours. This skin will be as clean as the blood that flows below it, for the condition of the skin reflects the condition of all that lies beneath it.

There are three layers of skin: the outer, inner and middle layers. The outer skin is the visible layer or "hide." The inner skin is called the **mucous membrane**. The middle skin (or **serous membrane**) lines the walls of the lungs, heart, abdomen and pelvic cavities, as well as those of the head and joints.

Notes

[1] Henry G. Bieler, M.D., *Food is Your Best Medicine*, Ballantine Books, 1965, p. 45.

[2] Cheryl Townsley, *Cleansing Made Simple*, LFH Publishing, 2001, p. 18.

[3] Ibid., p. 15.

Chapter Summary

Digestion of carbohydrates starts in the mouth through the secretion of the enzymes ptyalin and amylase from the salivary glands. Food travels then through the esophagus into the stomach. The stomach's churning and secretion of digestive juices converts the food to chyme. Pepsin and HCl from the stomach break down protein. Chyme then enters the duodenum, where bicarbonates and digestive enzymes from the pancreas neutralize stomach acid and break down food into its component parts. Bile is secreted from the gallbladder into the duodenum to emulsify fat and decompose it for distribution. Food residue passes next into the small intestine, where 90% of absorption takes place. It then enters the large intestine through the ileocecal valve, traveling up the ascending colon, across the transverse, down the descending colon, through the rectum and out the anus. Liquid and nutrients pass through the wall of the large intestine into the bloodstream, then on to the liver for processing and filtration.

The colon houses three types of bacteria: good, neutral and bad. A balance of approximately 80% good/neutral to 20% bad is desirable for health maintenance. This balance will assist the body in normal elimination of solid waste, a minimum of one daily bowel movement (preferably two to three).

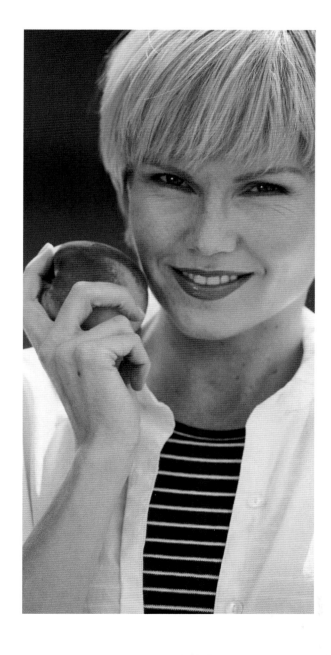

There are approximately 44.9 million visits annually to ambulatory care facilities due to diseases of the digestive system (1999).

Source:
National Center for Health Statistics; Advance Data 320, 321 and 322.

CHAPTER 2

IMPAIRED
digestion

Impaired digestion is the beginning of a process that ends with chronic disease (see figure 1). Throughout, there are many factors that can and do influence the process. Some of the factors are stress, drugs, alcohol, cigarettes, genetics, diet and environmental toxins. The only one not controlled easily in this process is genetics. A closer look at the digestive system reveals the effects of these influences.

Today there are over 100 million Americans who suffer from digestive disorders, making gastrointestinal complaints the third leading cause of illness in this country. In this chapter, we will examine the causes and clinical implications of impaired digestion. Ultimately, poor digestion will encourage the advancement of age-related illness and autoimmune diseases such as arthritis, fibromyalgia, chronic fatigue, irritable bowel syndrome and more.

Food must be in the proper form for the body to absorb it. For example, carbohydrates must be converted into a form of glucose, and protein into amino acids. If food is not converted properly, it will pass through the system in an undigested form and produce toxins. If these toxins are not promptly eliminated, they can lead to chronic disease. As figure 1 shows, impaired digestion is the beginning of a series of problems that lead ultimately to chronic disease. Many of these problems are part of our daily life:

• Stress
• Processed food consumption
• Inadequate chewing/excess fluid intake with meals
• Improper food-combining
• Overeating

When these factors affect our ability to properly digest and process foods, the results can include:

• Lowered production of hydrochloric acid (HCl)

2

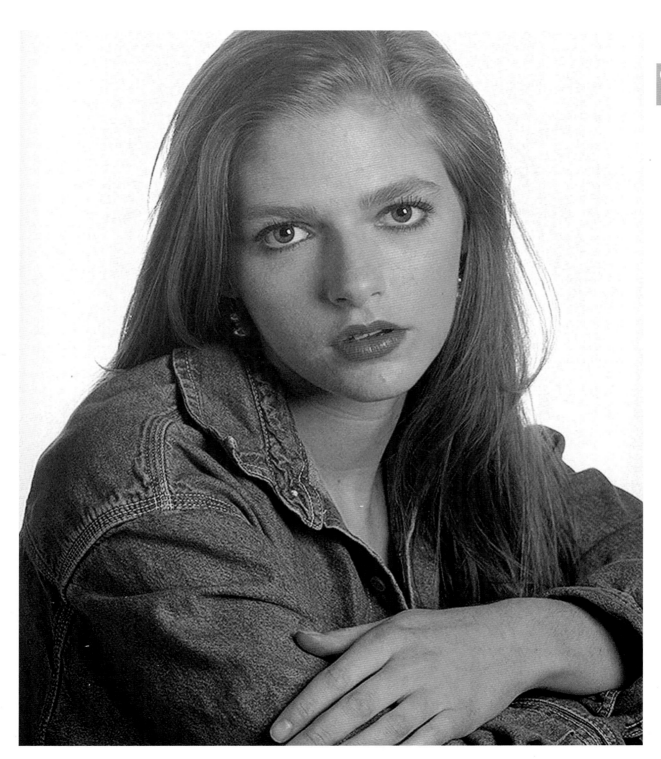

- Pancreatic impairment (reduced enzyme production)
- Imbalanced intestinal pH
- Food sensitivities

The following section explores these factors in more detail.

CAUSES OF POOR DIGSTION

The Role of Stress

There are several reasons why the body fails to digest food properly. A primary cause of poor digestion is stress. All unconscious activity in the body is controlled by the **autonomic nervous system**. The autonomic nervous system controls the digestive system and our reactions to stress. The body is designed to divert energy, blood, enzymes and oxygen away from the digestive organs when stress is experienced. If, for example, we have just eaten breakfast and are late for work, the body will support our mad dash through traffic before it will help digest a meal.

Any type of stress can have an adverse effect on the digestive process, virtually stopping it by lowering pancreatic enzyme production and inhibiting HCl production. Stress can be of a physical, mental or emotional nature.

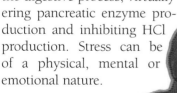

Physical stress is tangible. Infections (even low-grade, sub-clinical ones), as well as trauma from injuries and surgery, are obvious types of physical stress. Dietary indiscretions (such as high sugar intake)

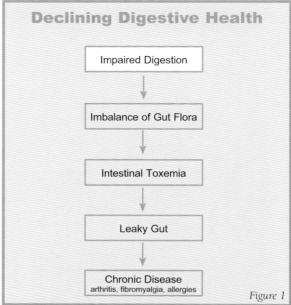

Declining Digestive Health

Impaired Digestion

↓

Imbalance of Gut Flora

↓

Intestinal Toxemia

↓

Leaky Gut

↓

Chronic Disease
arthritis, fibromyalgia, allergies

Figure 1

constitute another type of physical stress that can have an adverse effect on the digestive system. Less obvious are more minor physical stressors like noise pollution and minor injuries such as cuts and bruises.

Emotional and mental stress—including financial worries, unhappy home life, unfulfilled career aspirations and arguments—all are a strain on the physical body and adversely alter its physiology. Emotional stress causes the body to use its nutritional reserves. Once these nutritional reserves are depleted, digestion becomes impaired, owing to a lack of enzymes needed for the digestive process to function adequately. It's easy to see how any type of emotional or mental stress can become a digestive stress. It is extremely important to cultivate a relaxed state of mind when eating. This ensures unimpaired blood circulation needed for the organs of digestion to work properly.

In today's world, we're literally surrounded by environmental stress in the form of pollution, chemical additives and drugs. Pollutants are primarily man-made chemicals that don't belong in the body but have found their way there through contaminated air and water supplies. A growing number of these will pollute the environment and our bodies in the future, adding more stress to already overburdened systems.

> **There are more than 80,000 toxic chemicals in use today, with 1,200 new ones added annually.**

Chemicals also find their way into the body in the form of additives (approximately 5,000 of them) used to preserve, color, flavor, emulsify and otherwise treat our food. The ingestion of drugs, both prescription and non-prescription, adds more chemical stress. Even a simple visit to the dentist is likely to increase the toxic load on the body. The mercury and other metals in a "silver" filling can result in oral toxicity, which ultimately causes systemic toxicity. Excessive toxins (chemicals, pollution and drugs) in the body must be processed and removed. This detoxification process uses large amounts of energy, which leaves little energy for proper digestive function. Improper digestion, as noted, can ultimately lead to degenerative and chronic disease.

Processed Food Consumption

Processed foods are those that have been through a commercial refining process, which includes the application of high temperatures. Such processing serves the purpose of increasing shelf life. The down side is that it also destroys some nutrients, creating a situation of imbalance and deficiency.

Refined carbohydrates include all products made with white sugar and flour. During the refining process, these foods are stripped of dozens of essential nutrients, including trace minerals

needed for carbohydrate combustion. A steady diet of refined carbohydrates forces the body to rob itself of the chromium, manganese, cobalt, copper, zinc and magnesium needed to digest the carbohydrates. Once these minerals are depleted, the body is unable to digest carbohydrates properly (processed or natural). Consequently, these partially digested foods will **ferment** into simple sugars and alcohols, providing fuel for yeast and bacteria and leading to indigestion, gas and bloating, which increases the body's toxic load.

Regular intake of refined carbohydrates therefore increases both toxicity and deficiency, creating not only digestive disturbance but ultimately also serious health problems. Refined carbs feed the bad bacteria, irritate digestive organs and reduce the speed and efficiency of digestion.

Fiber is a non-nutritive food component that provides bulk to move food residue through the intestines. It is found naturally in whole grains, fruits and vegetables. When whole grains are milled, the bran and germ portions are discarded, and with them the fiber and many nutrients. Americans typically consume too little fiber and too many refined carbohydrates, and tend to eat inadequate amounts of fruits and vegetables. Lack of fiber results in a slow transit time of food through the digestive tract. According to Michael Murray, ND, the average daily fiber consumption in the U.S. is approximately 20 grams per person[1] (35-45 grams of fiber is needed daily). The result of such a low fiber intake is a transit time of more than 48 hours (more than twice what it should be). Such a slow transit time can result in the absorption of toxins from putrefied fecal material

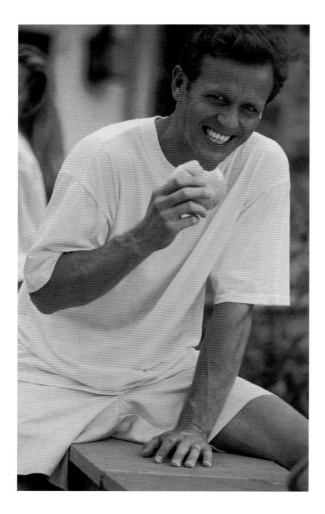

that has not been eliminated. The absorption of toxins from within the body's digestive system is a form of self-poisoning or "**autointoxication**," which can lead to degenerative disease.

The refining process has resulted in fragmentation, not only of grain products but also oil products. Virtually every oil product on supermarket shelves is refined, bleached and deodorized (and not so labeled). During refinement, processed oil products are often exposed to heat, light and oxygen, and are usually extracted with solvents such as hexane (a toxin)

to obtain higher yields. Thus much of the quality of the oils is lost in the refinement process.

Many oils are hydrogenated, which increases shelf life at a high cost to consumer health. This process involves the use of extremely high temperatures and super-saturation of the oil with hydrogen, using a nickel catalyst. **Hydrogenation** of oil results in the formation of unnatural "**trans**" **fatty acids** (TFAs), which constitute 50–60% of the fat content in commonly used "partially hydrogenated vegetable oils." Medical research has proven that human consumption of trans fats increases total cholesterol, **LDL** ("bad" cholesterol), and **lipoprotein a**, while decreasing **HDL** ("good" cholesterol), all of which increase the risk of heart disease. Approximately 70% of all the vegetable oils used in foods such as crackers, cookies, pastries, cakes, snack chips, imitation cheese, candies and fried foods contain several grams of trans fats.

Inadequate Chewing/Drinking with Meals

As previously noted, carbohydrate digestion begins in the mouth with the secretion of the enzyme ptyalin. This enzyme, mixed with saliva, is crucial to proper digestion of carbohydrates. Food chewed into small particles is then completely mixed with a saliva/enzyme mixture to begin digestion. When food is swallowed after only a few short chews, as so many of us busy people do, there is insufficient time for ptyalin to do its job. Consequently, carbohydrate digestion is impaired. Large, inadequately chewed food

> In addition to chewing food thoroughly, care should be taken to restrict fluid intake with meals, as over-consumption of liquids may dilute digestive enzymes and HCl, thus impairing digestion.

particles are harder for the body to digest and can result in gas, bloating and indigestion.

Improper Food-Combining

Of the many food-combining rules that have been proposed, two emerge as most important in terms of their impact on the greatest number of people. These two rules are: (1) *Eat fruits alone or leave them alone* (Fruit is most beneficial when eaten 20 to 30 minutes before other food.) and (2) *Do not combine proteins and starchy carbohydrates at the same meal.* Disregarding these rules can slow down digestion, resulting in much gas and bloating. Here's why: Fruit is digested very rapidly when eaten alone because it is not digested in the stomach but rather is pre-digested, being high in enzymes. Fruit (especially melons) passes through the stomach in a very short period of time, 20 to 30 minutes, releasing nutrients in the intestine. If eaten with (or after) other foods, then fruit will not be able to move through the digestive tract as rapidly as usual since other foods, especially proteins, have a much longer transit time. (Meat, for example, has a transit time of as much as six hours.) Fruit will ferment if eaten last since other foods will block its passage through the digestive tract. The result could be gastric distress.

Combining proteins (like meat) with heavy starches (like pasta or potatoes) may not pose a problem for a person with a strong digestive system; however, this combination places a heavy demand on the output of both proteolytic (protein-digesting) enzymes and amalse (starch-digesting), stressing the digestive system. Those with weak digestive systems may want to avoid these combinations. While separating proteins and starchy carbohydrates is desirable for those who have a slow **metabolism** (slow transit time), those who are **hyper-metabolic** (have a fast transit time)—about 20% of the population—will

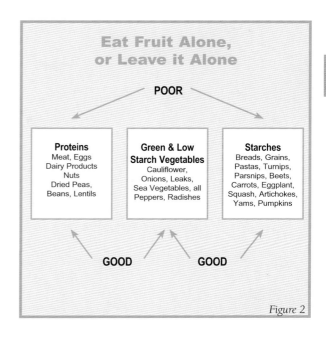

Figure 2

actually benefit from this combination because it will help to slow their metabolic rate.

These food-combining rules are most important to immune-compromised people with delicate digestive systems. Others, with good health, a hardy constitution and strong digestive organs may be able to disregard these rules without experiencing ill effects. It may be wiser therefore to view them as "guidelines" rather than "rules."

Over-Eating

Overindulging in even the most nutritious foods will reduce their benefits, for the body will be unable to use the nutrients. Today, there is a virtual epidemic of obesity due in large part, undoubtedly, to the nutrient deficiency of the Standard American Diet (SAD). Nutrient imbalances and deficiencies may cause people to select foods unwisely. Overeating may be largely the mind's unconscious effort to satisfy the body's hunger for the missing nutrients (lost during processing and preparation).

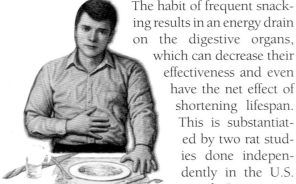

The habit of frequent snacking results in an energy drain on the digestive organs, which can decrease their effectiveness and even have the net effect of shortening lifespan. This is substantiated by two rat studies done independently in the U.S. and Germany in the early 1970s. "Both groups found the rats fed but once a day had a lower body weight and higher enzyme activities in the pancreas and fat cells. It was also found that the life-span of the controlled eaters was longer by 17%."[2]

CLINICAL IMPLICATIONS OF IMPAIRED DIGESTION

Low Production of Hydrochloric Acid

Hydrochloric acid (HCl) is a digestive acid produced in the stomach by millions of parietal cells—the cells that line the stomach. HCl is so strong that it will burn your skin. The lining of the stomach is protected from this acid however by a layer of mucus. Adequate production of HCl is critical to good health and a properly functioning digestive system because it:

- Triggers esophageal sphincter to close—keeping food and acid from refluxing
- Helps break down protein
- Sterilizes food by destroying bacteria and microbes that are present
- Is required for production of **intrinsic factor** (needed for B12 absorption)
- Is needed for mineral absorption
- Signals the pancreas to secrete enzymes in the small intestine

The secretion of HCl triggers the lower esophageal sphincter (LES) muscle to tighten after food enters the stomach. This is extremely important as the tightening of the LES keeps food and HCl from refluxing into the esophagus. Lower HCl production could contribute to a weakening of the LES and be a major contributing factor to reflux/GERD.

> **Some studies have found that 50% of the people older than 60 have low stomach acid.**

HCl is critical in the digestion of protein. It breaks apart the chains of amino acids (protein constituents, which look like strings of pearls). Its presence also signals the production of pepsin, a protein-splitting enzyme, which further ensures that the amino acids are split into shorter chains to complete the process.

Indigestion, heartburn and ulcers are often thought to be caused by an over-production of stomach acid (hydrochloric acid). This is a common misconception. There is very little correlation between stomach acid production and these common digestive symptoms. In other words, you may experience heartburn or indigestion if you produce too much or not enough stomach acid. What is troubling is that physicians often treat chronic indigestion and heartburn with drugs that lower production of stomach acid. In fact, the largest selling drug in America (and the world) is an acid reducing medication. While decreasing production of stomach acid may relieve the symptoms of indigestion and heartburn, this may worsen the condition in the long term. This is particularly true if the underlying cause of indigestion and heartburn is an under production of stomach acid. There are many studies that have found that as we age hydrochloric acid production decreases by as much as 50%. When we do not produce enough stomach acid to digest our foods, or we eat too much food at one sitting, heartburn and indigestion are often

Test Your pH

One way to determine if you have a HCl deficiency is to use special pH testing paper (which measures acidity/alkalinity) first thing in the morning to obtain a reading of the pH of your saliva. Record the number corresponding to the color change on the paper, and then test the saliva again about 1/2 hour after eating breakfast. You should see an increase in pH, ideally by two whole numbers (from a pH of 7 to a pH of 9, for example). If the second reading decreases instead of increases, and/or if the first reading was initially low (less than 6.5), it is an indication of a need for more stomach acid.[5]

Figure 3

the result. Prior to the 1960s, it was common for physicians to prescribe betaine hydrochloride (an acid) for cases of indigestion or heartburn. I have personally found this to be effective at relieving heartburn and indigestion. Until the mid-1990s, many physicians still believed that ulcers were caused by an over-production of stomach acid. It is now commonly known that the bacterium H. pylori is a common cause of stomach ulcers, and physicians now use antibiotics to treat ulcers. The message is clear. Hydrochloric acid is needed for adequate digestion of foods.

We constantly eat food that contains microbes. There is no way to know if food prepared and served at restaurants is properly washed or if the water is clean. So, when your HCl level is low, there is a greater possibility of parasitic infestation. Another problem that can occur when HCl levels are low is vitamin B12 deficiency. HCl aids in the production of intrinsic factor in the stomach. Intrinsic factor binds with extrinsic (from food) B12 to enable the absorption of B12 in the intestine. The lowering of stomach acid with age can inhibit the production of intrinsic factor and thus the absorption of B12. Many senior citizens have B12 deficiencies, which can result in muscle weakness and fatigue.

Other problems with low HCl include poor mineral absorption and reduced enzyme production. The presence of HCl in the duodenum signals the pancreas to release water, bicarbonate and enzymes. When the pH of the stomach is elevated or alkaline (due to HCl deficiency), the pH of the rest of the body can become imbalanced. The body cannot maintain homeostasis under these conditions, and serious degenerative diseases, including cancer, congestive heart failure, osteoporosis and Alzheimer's disease, may result.[3]

The symptoms of HCl deficiency are basically the same as those of excessive HCl production. These symptoms include:

- Bad breath
- A loss of taste for meat
- Stomach pain
- Fullness, distension in the abdomen
- Nausea/vomiting
- Gas
- Diarrhea and constipation
- Severe heartburn
- Intestinal parasites or abnormal flora
- Iron deficiency
- Itching around the rectum
- Undigested food in the stool
- Acne
- Candida infections
- Food allergies
- Weak, peeling and cracked fingernails[4]

Antacids…The Solution or the Problem?
When these symptoms are treated with antacids,

there may be initial relief, but more problems eventually result. Antacids inhibit the body's natural ability to produce HCI. As noted, HCI has many benefits, including sterilization of our food. Without enough HCl, uncontrolled growth of every kind of microorganism

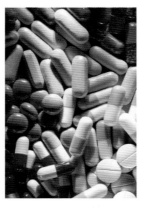

in the stomach such as yeast, fungi and bacteria can result. Antacids alkalize the lower stomach, triggering the release of more acid, requiring more antacids. A vicious cycle occurs, with the stomach alternating from too much acid production to not enough. This will eventually exhaust the cells of the stomach, and they will become unable to produce stomach acid.

Many antacids contain aluminum compounds, which can bind the bowels, accumulate in the brain and could be a factor in the eventual development of Alzheimer's disease. Aluminum-containing antacids can also cause long-term depletion of the calcium stored in the body, contributing to osteoporosis. Taking a medication for heartburn that could cause ulcers, create an overgrowth of yeast and bacteria, contribute to Alzheimer's disease and damage the bones in the body is not a good solution. A more natural approach to the problem of low HCl would be to take HCl supplements. More on that later.

Pancreatic Insufficiency

Besides secreting water and bicarbonates into the duodenum to neutralize the acidity of chyme, the pancreas also secretes enzymes, which break down carbohydrates, protein and fats. Enzymes that convert proteins (into amino acids) are the proteases. Part of the job of protease enzymes is to prevent allergic reactions resulting from the

absorption of non-digested protein, which causes an immune response in the lymphatic tissue of the intestinal tract. Fifty percent of the body's lymphatic tissue lines the intestinal tract to protect us from microbial invaders and toxins.

Poor production of pancreatic juice is termed **pancreatic insufficiency**. The condition can result from aging, physical and mental stress, nutritional deficiencies, a diet of only cooked foods, exposure to toxins or radiation, genetic weakness, drugs and infection. Low HCl production will also inhibit pancreatic secretions.

Pancreatic insufficiency is an underlying cause of high blood sugar (**hyperglycemia**). It is commonly found in people with **candidiasis** (an overgrowth of the yeast germ *Candida albicans*) and those with parasite infections. Symptoms of pancreatic insufficiency include gas, indigestion, abdominal discomfort, bloating, food sensitivities and the presence of undigested fat (and other food) in the stool.[5]

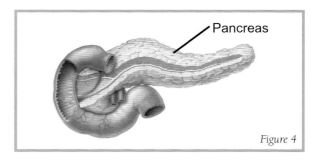

Pancreas

Figure 4

Lowered Enzyme Production

Enzymes are complex proteins that cause chemical changes in other substances. They are the basis of all metabolic activity in the body, facilitating more than 150,000 biochemical reactions and empowering every cell in the body to function. There are three types of enzymes in the body: **metabolic**, **digestive** and **food** enzymes. Metabolic enzymes run and heal the body, giving structure to **macronutrients** (fats, carbohydrates,

The Role of Digestive Enzymes

The Enzyme				
Protease	**Converts**	Proteins	**into**	Amino Acids
Lipase	**Converts**	Fat	**into**	Fatty Acids
Amylase	**Converts**	Carbohydrates	**into**	Sugars

Figure 5

protein) and repairing damage. The body cannot function or heal without metabolic enzymes. Digestive enzymes are manufactured by the pancreas. There are about 22 pancreatic enzymes, chief of which are protease (digests protein), lipase (for fat digestion) and amylase (for carbohydrate digestion). Food enzymes also digest food; however, they are supplied to the body solely through the diet, only from raw foods. These raw foods supply enzymes to digest the food in which they're found, with no extras to digest other foods.

Cooking at temperatures of more than 116 degrees destroys food enzymes. Enzyme deficiencies are widespread in the American culture because virtually all food in the standard diet is refined (heat has been applied during processing).

Imbalanced Intestinal pH

pH is a measurement of acidity/alkalinity. It is measured on a scale from 0 to 14, with substances becoming increasingly more alkaline as the number increases, as per the following table:

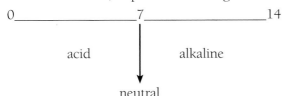

0 _____ 7 _____ 14

acid   alkaline

neutral

The optimal pH for digestion varies throughout the digestive tract as food moves through it. In the healthy digestive tract, the saliva secretes

Changing pH in the Body

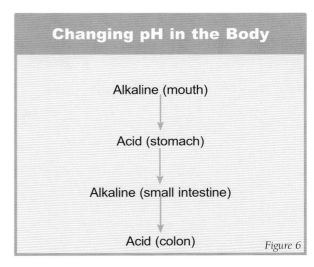

Alkaline (mouth)

↓

Acid (stomach)

↓

Alkaline (small intestine)

↓

Acid (colon)

Figure 6

alkaline juices into the mouth; the stomach produces acid secretions; the pancreas and gallbladder discharge alkaline juices to buffer the stomach acid; therefore, the small intestine is alkaline, and the colon is normally acid due to the presence of large populations of bacteria. So, there is a pH shift: alkaline (mouth) to acid (stomach) to alkaline (small intestine) to acid (colon).

An imbalance of intestinal **pH** can result from impairment of digestive secretions such as HCl and from pancreatic insufficiency. Lowered HCl production can result in an alkaline (rather than an acid) stomach. Pancreatic insufficiency could create an acidic (rather than an alkaline) environment in the small intestine if the pancreas fails to produce bicarbonate to alkalize the chyme leaving the stomach and entering the duodenum. Antacids can further complicate matters if taken habitually in an attempt to decrease heartburn.

If the pH of any of these key digestive organs is incorrect, the result will be incomplete digestion and its adverse health consequences.

Food Sensitivities

The improper digestion of food (especially proteins) can lead to an allergy-like response.

When undigested food particles enter the circulation through the walls of the intestine, the body responds as if they were foreign invaders, known as antigens. An immune attack begins with the body producing antibodies (chemical bullets), which bind to the antigens, forming what are known as **immune complexes**. When this occurs, there may be enough of an immune system imbalance to create indigestion. In addition, stress can create a **sympathetic dominance** (fight or flight syndrome), which impairs digestion. Both of these responses can increase intestinal permeability and lead to more **food sensitivities**.

As the breakdown of the digestive and elimination processes occurs, an adverse reaction to any food can result. Certain foods show up more often than others as "**allergens**." These include milk, soy, wheat, corn, yeast, sugar, eggs and the "**nightshade**" family, which consists of white potatoes, eggplant, tomatoes, chili peppers and garden peppers. Tobacco and certain drugs are also included in the nightshade category. Among the drugs so categorized are those containing atropine, belladonna and scopolamine, found in most sleeping pills.[6] It is important to know that a sensitivity or allergy to any food can develop, regardless of nutritional value or lack of it. It is also important to distinguish between an allergy and sensitivity.

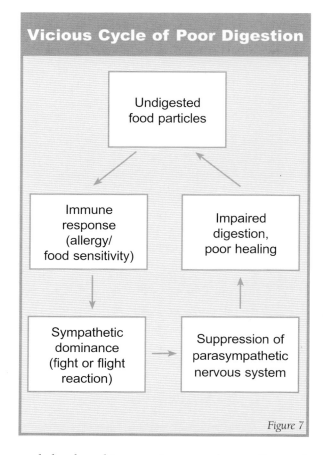

Vicious Cycle of Poor Digestion

Undigested food particles

Immune response (allergy/ food sensitivity)

Impaired digestion, poor healing

Sympathetic dominance (fight or flight reaction)

Suppression of parasympathetic nervous system

Figure 7

Food allergies are easy to recognize. They involve immediate, strong reactions to foods, whereas a sensitivity expresses itself in a much more subtle 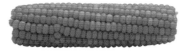 way. Food sensitivities are delayed reactions to foods, which can occur anywhere from a few hours to a few days after exposure. With the allergic response, the areas of the body affected by exposure to the allergen are generally limited to the air passages, skin and digestive tract. When someone eats strawberries

and develops hives, or is exposed to pollen and starts sneezing, this is a classic allergic response, the type for which allergists test with skin prick tests. This type of reaction is an IgE (immunoglobulin E) antibody–mediated reaction to antigens in the food. This is an acute **allergy**.

The IgG (as distinct from IgE) antibody reaction to food is generally known as a food sensitivity rather than a food allergy. The delayed food sensitivity, in contrast to the acute allergy, may affect any organ or tissue of the body, resulting in a wide array of physical and emotion- 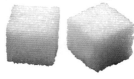 al symptoms. Such reactions, because they are delayed (by as much as three days), are frequently

Effects of the Sympathetic and Parasympathetic Systems on Selected Organs

Effector	Sympathetic System	Parasympathetic System
Pupils of eye	Dilation	Constriction
Sweat glands	Stimulation	None
Digestive glands	Inhibition	Stimulation
Heart	Increased rate and strength of beat	Decreased rate and strength of beat
Bronchi of lungs	Dilation	Constriction
Muscles of digestive system	Decreased contraction (peristalsis)	Increased contraction
Kidneys	Decreased activity	None
Urinary bladder	Relaxation	Contraction and emptying
Liver	Increased release of glucose	None
Penis	Ejaculation	Erection
Adrenal medulla	Stimulation	None
Blood vessels to:		
Skeletal muscles	Dilation	Constriction
Skin	Constriction	None
Respiratory system	Dilation	Constriction
Digestive Organs	Constriction	Dilation

Chart taken from *The Human Body in Health and Disease* by Memmler, Cohen, Wood, p. 148

Figure 8

not recognized as food sensitivities. It is common for reactive foods to be consumed frequently, to the point of addiction. By consuming such foods habitually, the body (unconsciously) avoids withdrawal symptoms. Unfortunately, this also perpetuates digestive disorders. When sensitive foods are eaten daily, the small intestine responds to the offenders by producing an antibody/antigen response. With the passing of time, this response irritates the digestive lining by producing inflammation. The response is analogous to wearing wool every day against the outer skin. The skin would eventually react by becoming inflamed. The same holds true for the lining of the gut.

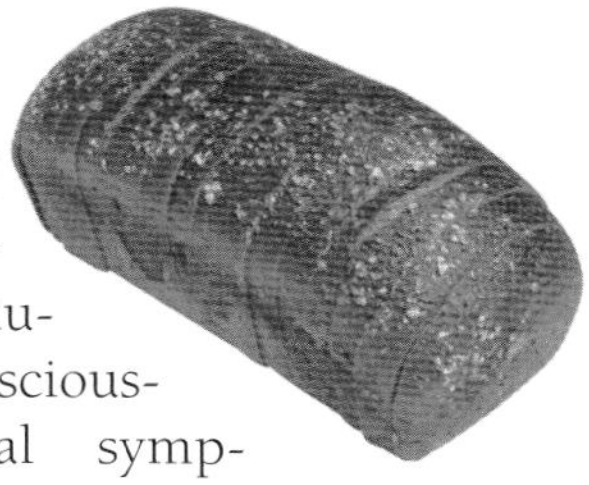

If people avoid the foods to which they're sensitive, they may start to feel somewhat better, but if digestion isn't improved, they will develop new sensitivities. On the other hand, if digestion is improved and toxins eliminated, sensitivities and allergies will be decreased or eliminated.

Both sensitivities and allergies may develop in response to anything in the environment—not just food. The response to the antigen—be it corn or petrochemicals—can affect any organ of the body. The gut will always be involved, however. Poor digestion is both the cause and the ultimate result of the allergic response or sensitivity, as figure 7 indicates. Significant stress will definitely lead to sympathetic dominance (see figure 8). This decreases digestive efficiency (less enzymes, etc.) and increases intestinal permeability, setting the stage for food allergies or sensitivities. The more food allergies or sensitivities, the more reactive the immune system becomes, creating more and more circulating antigen/antibody complexes. These will promote inflammation throughout the body, especially in the GI tract, creating further problems.

With food allergies and sensitivities, there is an element of increased permeability (leaky gut) of the intestinal tract that plays a dominant role in initiating the process. Undigested food particles have the effect of initiating an immune response, (allergic reaction) when they have made their way into the bloodstream. This can occur only when the lining of the intestine becomes porous. This condition of increased permeability or porosity of the lining of the intestine is known as **"leaky gut syndrome."**

Notes

[1] Michael Murray, N.D., *The Healing Power of Foods*, Prima Publishing, 1993, p. 83.

[2] Dr. Edward Howell, *Enzyme Nutrition*, Avery Publishing Group, Inc., 1985, p. 112.

[3] Judy Kitchen, "Hypochlorhydria: A Review – Part I," *Townsend Letter for Doctors and Patients*, October 2001, p. 56.

[4] Ibid., p. 58.

[5] Elizabeth Lipski, M.S., C.C.N., *Digestive Wellness*, Keats Publishing, Inc., 1996, p. 207.

[6] James Braly, M.D., *Dr. Braly's Food Allergy and Nutrition Revolution*, Keats Publishing, Inc., p. 437.

Chapter Summary

Stress, broadly defined as anything that causes an extra load on the body, can be viewed as the cause of digestive dysfunction. Digestive stress comes in many forms, which may include:

- Emotional or physical stress
- Poor diet
- Medications
- Environmental toxins
- Over-consumption of processed food

If stress from any of these sources continues for an extended period of time, the result is a burdened digestive system and stressed supporting organs (such as liver and pancreas). The end result is altered function or structure of the body's organ systems, which develops into:

- **Deficiency of HCl**, needed to break down proteins and protect from harmful microorganisms
- **Pancreatic insufficiency** (reduced enzyme and bicarbonate secretion), a precursor to more serious disease
- **Imbalanced intestinal pH**, which prevents proper digestion of foods due to excessive acidity or alkalinity of digestive juices
- **Food sensitivities and allergies**, which can be both the cause and the result of poor digestion

All of these stressors impair the digestive process, which leads to an imbalance of gut flora, intestinal toxemia, candida and parasites, leaky gut and chronic disease.

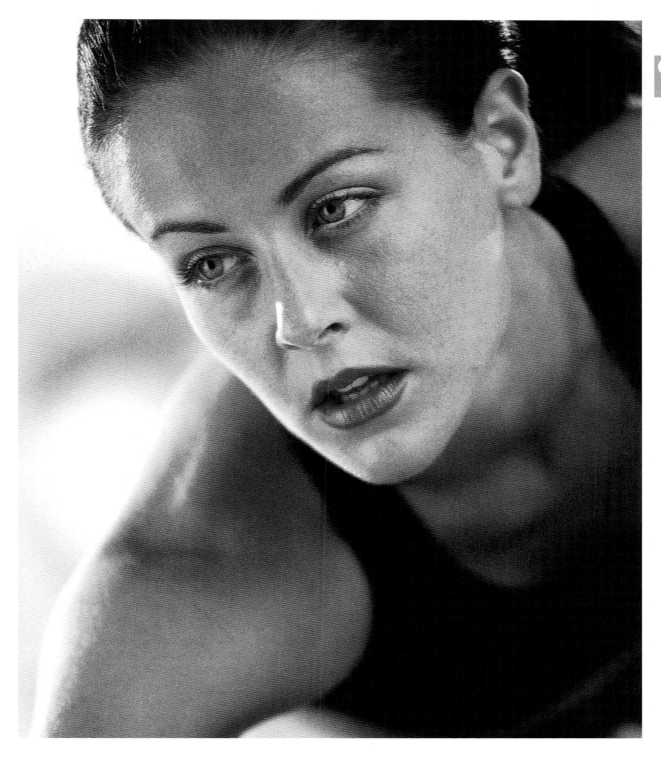

CHAPTER 3

EFFECTS OF
digestive DYSFUNCTION

Approximately half of the population carries at least one form of parasite. Twenty-five percent of these people have an active infection with symptoms.

Source:
The Parasite Menace,
by Skye Weintraub, M.D.

IMBALANCE OF GUT FLORA

The micro flora composition of the intestinal tract is complex. There are approximately 500 different species of micro flora that are part of the normal intestinal environment. There is a simple way to understand the different bacteria groupings in the gut: In every individual there is a ratio of **good** (health-promoting) bacteria, **neutral** bacteria (**commensal**) and **pathogenic** (disease-causing) bacteria. All of these organisms are competing for food and space in the digestive tract.

It is important that the good bacteria be abundant in the digestive tract. When the microbial population becomes incorrectly balanced, parasitic bacteria dominate. For example, if candida (which is a natural inhabitant of the gut) or some other microbe grows out of control, the body is in a state of **dysbiosis**. Dysbiosis (out of harmony or "disturbed biology") is a term coined by Dr. Eli Metchnikoff early in the twentieth century to describe an imbalance of intestinal flora and the accompanying conditions. Metchnikoff discovered the health benefits of probiotics and won the Nobel Prize in 1908 for his work with Lactobacilli. He theorized that toxic compounds produced by bacterial breakdown of food were the cause of degenerative disease and a major factor in aging. Beneficial flora are required for bacterial **fermentation** of dietary fiber, which results in **short-chain fatty acid** production. The short-chain fatty acids butyrate, acetate and lactate, support the production of new cells, which is vital in rebuilding the intestinal tract. Where dysbiosis is present, the intestinal wall cannot be rebuilt, as it normally would be, every three to five days. An extra benefit of the short-chain fatty acids is the prevention of colon cancer.

Many factors cause dysbiosis, including poor diet, slow transit time and emotional stress. Chemicals and certain

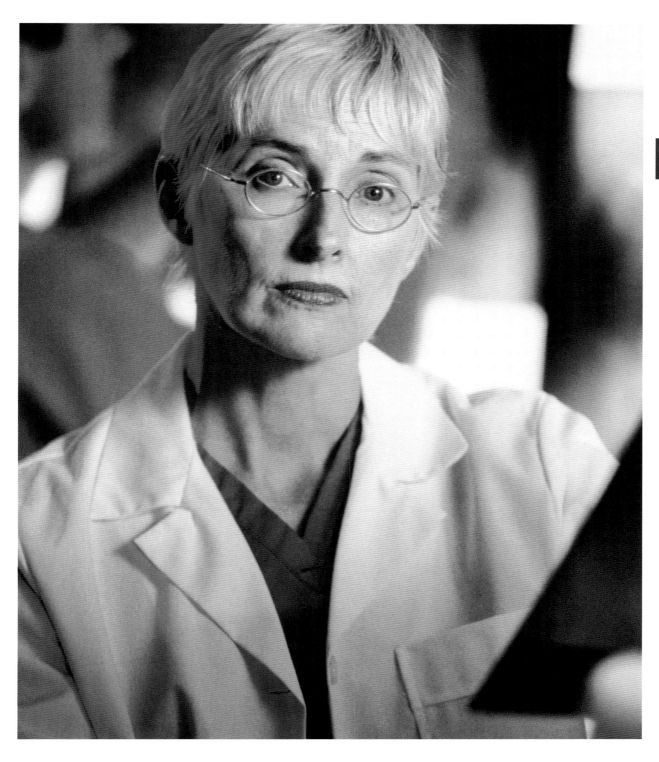

Good bacteria aids in:

- **Digestion of food**
- **Absorption of nutrients**
- **Production of B vitamins**
- **Production of antibodies**
- **Destruction of competing bacteria**

drugs can cause the condition, as can surgery and improper ileocecal valve (ICV) functioning. The ICV is the valve between the small intestine and large intestine. It is usually kept closed to prevent **reflux** (back flow) of fecal contents into the small intestine. Problems arise when constipation is present. As the peristaltic colonic waves attempt to propel the stool toward the rectum, backward pressure will push some of the liquid stool in the colon back through the ICV, causing contamination and colonization of the small intestine with colonic bacteria. This is medically known as "small bowel dysbiosis," a major cause of leaky gut syndrome. In addition, like the entire intestinal tract, the ICV muscular tone is controlled by the autonomic nervous system. When this system is imbalanced, a decrease in smooth muscle tone of the ICV could result in

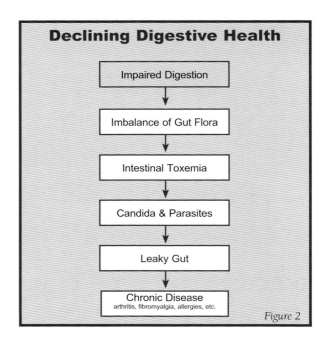

Figure 2

backflow of the colonic contents into the small intestine, again promoting leaky gut syndrome. Manipulation of autonomic nervous system balance may be helpful in providing normal intestinal tract tone and function. Modalities such as acupuncture, chiropractic manipulation, yoga and tai chi can be very helpful in this regard. The mechanics of the ICV and the recto-sigmoid portion of the colon can become compromised when the body is in the incorrect position for elimination of bowel contents. The correct posture would be a squatting position, which is the elimination posture used in much of the world.

Where dysbiosis is present, the ideal ratio of beneficial to putrefactive (pathogenic) bacteria (80:20) is upset, even reversed. When **putrefactive** bacteria proliferate in the intestinal tract, peristalsis becomes sluggish. This inhibition of muscular contractions in the cecum causes food residues to concentrate in the appendix where they stagnate and cause inflammation (appendicitis = inflammation of the appendix).

Causes of Intestinal Flora Imbalance

- Antibiotic use
- Refined carbohydrates
- Birth control pills
- Poor digestion/ elimination
- Stress
- Low fiber diet
- Steroid drug use
- X-rays/radiation therapy
- Chlorinated water
- Mercury toxicity
- Pollution

Figure 1

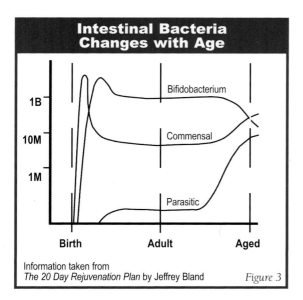

Intestinal Bacteria Changes with Age

Information taken from
The 20 Day Rejuvenation Plan by Jeffrey Bland

Figure 3

There are many aspects of today's lifestyles that contribute to the destruction of beneficial flora, leading to dysbiosis (see figure 1). Dysbiosis commonly occurs due to faulty digestion, which results in partially digested food reaching the end of the small intestine and entering the colon. The action of the colonic bacteria on partially digested food can result in the putrefaction of proteins and fermentation of carbohydrates, which may cause further growth of the pathogenic bacteria. This problem is greatly compounded when food stays in the intestinal tract too long (constipation).

INTESTINAL TOXEMIA

Intestinal toxemia, poisoning of the intestines, occurs when the bacteria present in the gut act upon undigested food. This interaction can produce toxic chemicals and gases. These toxins, in turn, can damage the mucosal lining, resulting in increased intestinal permeability (leaky gut). The net result is that the toxins are then able to spread throughout the body via the bloodstream. In the words of Dr. John Matsen, N.D., "If you don't digest your food quickly, some microorganisms will digest it for you, making toxins."[1] The

waste products from these microorganisms produce some extremely potent toxins, 78 known types, including skatoles, indols, phenols, alcohol, ammonia, acetaldehyde and formaldehyde.[2] All of these are examples of **endotoxins**, internally produced toxins. They are just as damaging to the body as external environmental toxins, **exotoxins**.

Intestinal toxins can also produce **free radicals**, molecules with unpaired electrons, which cause damage to cells when they rip electrons out of cell membranes. Free radicals live only momentarily, but can do a great amount of damage in that short period of time. Large numbers of free radicals are produced by dozens of intestinal toxins. When the body is unable to buffer against them due to toxic overload, disease results. To inactivate free radicals, the body deploys **antioxidants**, nutrients that act as free radical scavengers. Vitamins A, C and E and the minerals selenium and zinc are well known antioxidants. What is not so well known is that bile has even stronger free radical scavenging effects. This makes proper liver and gallbladder function important in preventing free radical damage.

In the beginning stages of intestinal toxemia, the body generally has sufficient nutritional reserves to manage the stress. At this point, it is not acutely distressed and may be without symptoms. However, as time passes, and the opportunistic

Drugs That Disrupt Intestinal Ecology

- Antibiotics
- Birth control pills
- Cortisone
- NSAIDs (non-steroidal anti-inflammatory drugs like ibuprofen)

Figure 4

organisms (bacteria, viruses, fungi, etc.) multiply, their toxic waste products overwhelm the body's defenses, transferring power from the "good" to the "bad guys." As this happens, organisms that normally inhabit the GI tract in smaller numbers, without causing harm, such as parasites and the yeast germ candida, can proliferate and produce symptoms such as gas, bloating, constipation, diarrhea, skin disorders, brain fog, chronic fatigue, irritable bowel syndrome and joint and muscle pain. These symptoms may or may not be recognized as the result of digestive stress, for they can occur anywhere in the body.

CANDIDA AND PARASITES— SECONDARY TOXIC SUPPRESSORS

Candida albicans, a yeast germ that becomes a problem when it proliferates and mutates to a fungal form, is actually a form of parasite, as are the other "critters" that normally inhabit the GI tract—microorganisms like viruses, bacteria, worms, amoebas and protozoa. These are all considered "secondary" toxic suppressors because of their opportunistic nature. They proliferate when the opportunity arises as a result of a shift in the body's terrain or internal environment (chang-

es in pH, microbial population, muscular tone, etc.). Such a shift results in energetic and chemical imbalance, and may be caused by impaired digestion. The shift in terrain can also result from environmental pollution and drugs. Drugs and environmental toxins (non-steroidal anti-inflammatory drugs [NSAIDs], chemicals, solvents, metals, etc.), coupled with structural misalignments and emotional stress, may be viewed as primary toxic suppressors, in that they create an environment for the secondary toxic suppressors—the opportunistic microorganisms, which include candida and parasites—to proliferate.

Candida and Other Fungi

Candida albicans is one of over 80 species of candida and more than 250 species of yeast, many of which are parasitic in the human body. Candida is normally present in the intestinal tract in small amounts. When it remains in yeast form and exists in balance with the trillions of bacteria that normally inhabit the digestive tract, all is well with the body's internal ecosystems. The ideal ratio of candida to bacteria is 1:1 million; that is, 1 yeast to 1 million bacteria. This critical balance will be maintained if:

• The immune system is functioning normally.

Profile of a Killer Disease

Egypt, 1924: British egyptologist, Hugh Evelyn-White, was among the first to enter the tomb of King Tutankhamen, shortly after its discovery in 1922 near the ruins of Luxor. Evelyn-White became one of the dozen explorers to die soon after visiting the site. "I have succumbed to a curse," wrote he in his own blood in 1924, moments before hanging himself. At the time no one could explain his suicide nor the many other mysterious deaths of other unfortunate ones who had entered the tomb. Coming primarily to look for gold and treasures, the excavators paid no attention to the pink, gray and green patches of fungi on the chamber walls. So, in reality, King Tut's curse was a really severe allergic reaction to fungi: fruits and vegetables placed in the tomb to feed the pharaoh throughout eternity but which, decaying over centuries, had created deadly molds.

- from *Candida* by LucDe Schepper, M.D., Ph.D., Lic. Ac., D.I. Hom, C. Hom.

- An optimal ratio of "good"/neutral to "bad" bacteria (80:20) is maintained.
- The pH of the colon is balanced (on the slightly acid side).

The medical community's awareness of candida has been largely limited to the local effects of acute infection (candidiasis). Such infection involves invasion of the mucous membranes, typically on the skin, in the mouth ("**thrush**") and in the vagina ("yeast" infection). A chronic overgrowth of candida in the intestines leads to an actual change in the form and function of the organism: It mutates from its yeast-like state to a fungal form. As such, candida can lead to a variety of conditions that can affect the body physically and mentally—a fact not well recognized or accepted in traditional medical circles.

While many physicians still treat a vaginal yeast infection as a localized problem, a growing number are becoming aware that such infection is invariably accompanied by an overgrowth of candida in the gut. To successfully resolve vaginal yeast problems and prevent their return, it is necessary to restore healthy conditions in the intestinal tract.

In its fungal state, candida grows very long roots, **rhizoids**, which actually puncture the mucous lining of the intestine. It also secretes acid, which can change the intestinal pH and can cause wear to this protective mucous lining. The resulting increased intestinal permeability

is known as leaky gut syndrome. This condition permits the entrance of the fungus (and its toxic waste products) into the bloodstream along with other foreign substances and undigested food particles. This leads to a series of problems discussed in the "Leaky Gut" section of this chapter.

Among the fungal toxins that can enter the bloodstream through the bowel wall is **acetaldehyde**, the major waste product produced by candida. Acetaldehyde is a poison that is converted by the liver into alcohol. As alcohol increases (due to insufficient oxygen in body tissues), symptoms associated with drunkenness develop: disorientation, dizziness and mental confusion. The poisonous effects of alcohol can result in anxiety, depression, irritability, headaches and fatigue. Acetaldehyde is just one of the candida toxins involved in enzyme destruction, which results in impaired detoxification ability, decreased cellular energy production and a release of cell-damaging free radicals. There are thought to be more than 100 such toxins produced by candida.

Candida toxins, carried to the liver by the bloodstream, proceed from there to other organs of the body—the brain, nervous system, joints, skin, etc. If the liver's detoxification ability is impaired due to inadequate nutrition and toxic overload, these toxins will be stored and can initiate chronic illness,

Conditions That May Arise From Fungal Toxins

- Chronic fatigue
- Depression and anxiety
- Infertility
- Miscarriage
- Skin problems
- Arthritis
- Intestinal disorders
- Digestive problems
- Migraine headaches
- Sugar cravings
- Nutritional deficiencies due to malabsorption
- Hormone imbalances
- Jock itch
- Fingernail/toenail fungus
- Insomnia
- ADD
- Interstitial cystitis
- Respiratory disorders
- Fibromyalgia
- Heart conditions
- Multiple Sclerosis
- Female problems
- Allergies and environmental sensitivities
- Bladder infections
- Prostatitis
- Blurred vision
- Athlete's foot
- Ringworm
- Bad breath

Figure 5

including those conditions listed in figure 5.

Fungal toxins, known as **mycotoxins**, suppress immune function. Some of these toxins, like **aflatoxin**, have been linked to cancer and hardening of the arteries.

Of special interest to women is a mycotoxin called **zearalenone**, which mimics the effects of estrogen in the body. It is produced by a mold, **fusarium graminearum**, and is found primarily in corn products, bananas and in the meat of cattle fed contaminated corn. An overabundance of estrogen can result in such health problems as fibroids, breast lumps, infertility and cancer. The presence of zearalenone in the body can cause these problems as well. There are currently no limits placed on the amount of this mycotoxin permitted in grains intended for human consumption.[3]

Although the food supply is monitored for the presence of common mycotoxins, it is not uncommon for molds to contaminate grains and more commonly to affect nuts. Fungus is, in fact, ubiquitous in the environment—that is, found virtually everywhere. It is in the air and food. It even exists on exposed surfaces and can quite literally "get under the skin." Its presence in the skin appears to be aggravated by use of alkaline soaps.[4] Exposure to moldy environments can result in fungi and their toxins being introduced into the body. Fungal infections can also be transmitted sexually.

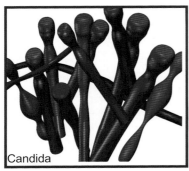

Candida

As previously mentioned, the presence of a small amount of yeast in the intestinal tract is normal, even helpful. However, it is abnormal for fungi to live inside the human body. Once inside, they live by ingesting dead or decaying matter.[5] Because fungal parasites must have sugar in order to survive, we often experience sugar cravings when harboring fungi. Giving in to those cravings only promotes more fungi.

Ironically, conditions that are caused by fungi are often medically treated with drugs (antibiotics, birth control pills, NSAIDs, cortisone) that destroy beneficial flora, thereby allowing fungi to proliferate, making the condition worse.

These drugs alter the terrain of the bowel by causing the extermination of good bacteria as well as bad. Any hormonal therapy, such as estrogen replacement, can cause an overgrowth of candida in this manner. The elevation of progesterone during pregnancy and in the second half of every menstrual cycle may also stimulate candida growth.

Candida secretes **carbon dioxide**, which may lead to gas and bloating. It is significant that poor digestion, which began the chain of events that led to candida overgrowth, can also be an effect of it. Many people are caught in this vicious cycle. **It is very important that those with candida overgrowth adhere to a special diet for a period of time, a diet free of sugar, starchy carbohydrates and fermented foods. Those who experience some of the described symptoms should complete the adult or children's candida self-analysis in the Appendix.**

Special laboratory tests for candida are available through aware physicians. These tests include candida antibody panels, intestinal permeability studies and digestive stool analysis. The International Health Foundation is a source for the names of physicians who are familiar with testing for and treating chronic systemic candida infection. The Foundation's services are available at 901-660-7090 (www.yeastconnetion. com). This non-profit organization, founded by pioneering candida researcher/doctor, William G. Crook, MD, offers publications to direct people to health care professionals who are interested in yeast-related health problems.

Most nutritional practitioners know about candida and the havoc it can create in the body. What isn't as well known is that candida infections often accompany parasite infections. The drain on the immune system by the parasite creates the opportunity for the candida to pro-liferate. The following section explains the effect parasite infection can have on human health.

Parasites

Parasites have become a dominant health problem that many believe has reached epidemic propor-tions. It's something of a *silent* epidemic, however, because the problem is likely to go undiagnosed or be misdiagnosed. Some parasite problems have been recognized, even made headlines— like the 1993 outbreak of **cryptosporidiosis** (caused by *cryptosporidium parvus*, a microscopic

---

Parasite Survey Facts

- More than half the people with infection had traveled overseas in the past five years.
- People traveling to Mexico and Europe had the highest risk of infection.
- People living in households where someone was infected had twice the risk of infection.
- Of people infected, some had no symptoms.
- Some people unknowingly acted as carriers. (Since there are no symptoms, they could have been unaware, been untreated and passed parasites on to others.)
- People infected by more than one parasite had similar symptoms to those with single infections.
- Women were twice as likely to be infected as men and were more heavily infected.
- The most prevalent pathogens were *E. histolytica*, *Giardia lamblia* and *Blastocystis hominis*.[7]

Figure 6

Parasite News

Instead of experiencing better health, most of the people living in North America are deterio-rating. People may be living longer, but they are not living healthier. There are many factors that contribute to this decline in health, but parasites may be one of the most overlooked.

The founding editor of *Prevention Magazine*, J.I. Rodale, once wrote an editorial stating that only those who protect themselves from the steadily increasing burden of toxic envi-ronmental pollution would survive in coming times.

---

parasite, found in the Milwaukee water supply), which made 400,000 people ill and killed 40. In that same year, parasite contamination was found in one out of every four municipal water supplies in 14 states. *Cryptosporidium* was featured on "ABC News" in the following year in reports that it had invaded New York City's water supply.

Another water-born parasite, **Giardia lamblia**, has been estimated by the Center for Disease Control to affect between 100,000 and 1 million people each year. In 1976, one of every six people in the U.S. was infected with one or more parasites.

In 1996, Dr. Omar Amin from Diagnostic Labs conducted a survey of 644 stool samples. In more than half (378), parasites were detected.[6] In the group, a number of typical characteristics emerged as shown in figure 6.

Parasites are difficult to detect. They tend to hide in the lining of the intestines, and they live in other organs as well. If parasites are in the heart or lungs, they will not appear in the stool regardless of how well it's analyzed! Some of the reasons parasites are difficult to recognize and diagnose:

- Parasitic infestation has generally been considered a disease of the tropics, so a doctor isn't likely to consider it when making a diagnosis.
- Parasitology is seldom presented in mainstream medical journals or medical schools.
- Other than records of the Center for Disease Control, there is little tracking for parasites. With lack of information and little training, doctors aren't apt to look for parasites as an underlying cause of illness. If the symptoms aren't confined to the digestive tract, parasitic infestation could surely go undiagnosed.

Symptoms of Parasites

- Constipation/diarrhea
- Digestive complaints (gas, bloating, cramps)
- Irritability/nervousness
- Irritable bowel syndrome
- Persistent skin problems
- Granulomas (tumor-like masses that encase destroyed larva or parasite)
- Overall fatigue
- Disturbed sleep
- Anemia
- Muscle cramps
- Joint pain
- Post nasal drip
- Teeth grinding
- Prostatitis
- Sugar cravings & ravenous appetite
- Allergies

Figure 7

Parasite Sources

- Contaminated raw fruits and vegetables
- Raw or rare meat
- Polluted water/tap water
- Pets
- Vectors (carriers, like mosquitoes)
- Through the skin
- Through the nose (inhaled)
- Restaurant dining (especially at salad and sushi bars)
- Camping
- Previous parasite infection/reinfection
- Working in infant care
- Travel
- Solvents, like prophyl alcohol (alter internal terrain, making it suitable for parasites)
- Contact with someone who has parasites (a carrier)

Figure 8

Parasites have a complex life cycle. Three of the most prevalent parasites found in the United States and worldwide shed at irregular intervals. This means that a parasite might be in the stool two to four days a week but not the rest of the week. If the person is tested for a parasite on a day it is not present, there will be a negative test result. The person would then go untreated. Therefore, it would be best for repeat stool samples (at least two to three) to be taken on nonconsecutive days.

Another difficulty with parasite detection is there are many newly identified parasites that have not been sufficiently studied or recognized as pathogenic. An example would be **cyclospora**, which was classified as a human parasite just a few years ago. The result of a parasite test done prior to the time that cyclospora was recognized as pathogenic would have been reported as negative even though cyclospora was present. By the 1990's, *Dientamoeba fragilis* was considered a pathogenic parasite though it had previously not been. The field of parasitology is thus evolving and continuously making discoveries of "new bugs." How do parasites threaten human health? They can injure the tissue of the digestive tract or most other organs. Most people don't realize this, but it is not only the parasite that can cause damage to the body, but also the waste that the parasite discharges into the body. This is part of the life cycle of any living organism: Food is ingested; waste is expelled. Parasites can disrupt the digestive process of the host, interfering with enzyme production and the breakdown of food. A properly functioning digestive system is critical to good health, so anything that disrupts this process will also affect the immune system. Remember: The mission of the parasite is to survive.

Degenerative disease can be associated with parasites. They create a mucous overlay in the gut that blocks absorption of nutrients so that the food we eat nourishes them, not us. Parasites can affect tissue anywhere in the body. Disorders that have been associated with parasites include arthritis, multiple sclerosis, appendicitis, both overweight and underweight conditions, cancer and epilepsy. Some cases of epilepsy have been associated with 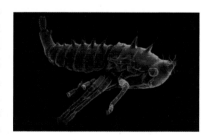 pork tapeworm. This is probably due to autoantibody production by the immune system in response to the parasites and the toxins they liberate. Pork should not be cooked in a microwave oven, as microwaves do not kill the **trichinella** worm in it.

Parasites can get into the blood and travel to any organ, causing problems that are often not recognized as parasite-related. Consequently, disorders involving parasites are often wrongly diagnosed. A roundworm infestation in the stomach can give the appearance of a peptic ulcer. Amoebic colitis can be mistaken for ulcerative colitis. Tapeworms can be the unsuspected cause of blood sugar disorders, both **hypoglycemia** and diabetes. Their eggs, when present in the liver, can be mistaken for cancer. Those parasites that fall into the **protozoa** category can cause arthritis-like pain, as well as leukemia-like symptoms. Chronic Giardia can be an undetected element or missing diagnosis in both candidiasis and chronic fatigue syndrome.

The appendix has been described as the "region of worms." Due to its location at the bottom of the cecum, food residues and waste tend to accumulate and stagnate there, producing conditions favorable for parasites to thrive and appendicitis to develop.

Medical texts don't contain much information about parasites other than stating they can cause diarrhea and malabsorption. It is important to bear in mind, however, that parasites can mimic other disorders and/or produce no noticeable symptoms. When they do cause symptoms, a wide range can be displayed, as indicated in figure 7.

Another factor that no doubt contributes to the growing parasite epidemic is the widespread use of drugs that suppress immunity as a side effect. Many of the drugs in common use today are immunosuppressive and therefore increase our susceptibility to parasitic infection.

Although many external factors contribute to the parasite problem (see figure 8), by far the biggest factor is an internal one—a dirty colon, largely the result of an unwholesome lifestyle and bacterial imbalance in the colon.

LEAKY GUT

Toxic irritation of the gut lining is step three in our flow chart in figure 1. Intestinal toxemia is the direct result of impaired digestion and imbalanced bacteria caused by numerous stressors. This toxemia occurs when the bacteria that line the walls of the intestinal mucosa act upon undigested food. The toxins produced from this interaction attack the delicate intestinal mucosa, and allow for the development of systemic candidiasis and parasitic infection. Repeated attacks by these internally produced toxins (endotoxins) will, as time passes, erode the gut lining. This is the basic mechanism by which leaky gut develops. It can also be caused or aggravated by a number of other factors, as indicated in figures 10 and 11.

According to Elizabeth Lipski, MS, CCN, "NSAIDs (non-steroidal anti-inflammatory drugs) can cause irritation and inflammation of the intestinal tract, leading to **colitis** and relapse of ulcerative colitis … [They] can cause bleeding and

Factors Leading to Leaky Gut

- Alcohol (gut irritant)
- Caffeine (gut irritant)
- Parasites (introduced into the body by contaminated food and water)
- Bacteria (introduced into the body by contaminated food and water)
- Chemicals (in processed foods)
- Enzyme deficiencies (e.g. celiac disease; lactase deficiency, causing lactose intolerance)
- Diet of refined carbohydrates ("junk" food)
- Prescriptive hormones (like birth control pills)
- Mold and fungal mycotoxins (in stored grains, fruit and refined carbohydrates)

Figure 10

ulceration of the large intestine and may contribute to complications of **diverticular disease** [outpouching of a segment of the intestine]."[8] Prolonged use of NSAIDs blocks the body's natural ability to repair the intestinal lining and also interferes with the production of prostaglandins, regulatory messengers that circulate throughout the body. The mucous lining of the small intestine is a semipermeable membrane that allows nutrients to enter the bloodstream, while shielding it from unwanted toxins and undigested food. This mucous lining is like the screen on a window in a house that

Unhealthy Digestive Tract

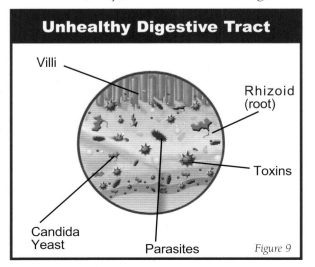

Villi

Rhizoid (root)

Toxins

Candida Yeast

Parasites

Figure 9

Drugs That Cause Leaky Gut

- NSAIDs (Non-steroidal anti-inflammatory drugs such as ibuprofen & aspirin)
- Antacids
- Steroids (includes prescription corticosteroids such as prednisone)
- Antibiotics

Figure 11

Autoimmune Diseases Resulting from Leaky Gut

- Lupus
- Rheumatoid arthritis
- Multiple sclerosis
- Chronic fatigue syndrome
- Fibromyalgia
- Crohn's disease
- Vasculitis
- Urticaria (hives)
- Raynaud's disease

- Alopecia areata
- Polymyalgia rheumatica
- Sjogren's syndrome
- Thyroiditis
- Vitilego
- Ulcerative colitis
- Diabetes

Figure 12

lets the air in but keeps the bugs out. It is also like the skin, in that it sloughs off a layer of cells naturally every three to five days and produces new cells to keep the lining semi-permeable. Once endotoxins have eroded this membrane, however, it becomes permeable. (The "screen" on the "window" becomes filled with holes!) Now the toxins and food particles, which would normally not be permitted to enter the system, literally leak into the bloodstream. The body then becomes confused and attacks these unwanted toxins, as if they were foreign substances, and develops antibodies (chemical bullets) against them.

CHRONIC DISEASE

The net result of the above process is development of **autoimmune disease**, where the body makes antibodies against its own tissues. There are some 80 recognized autoimmune diseases (see figure 12 for a partial list); the cause of all of them is "unknown" in medical circles.

Physicians are becoming increasingly aware of the importance of the GI tract in the development of autoimmune disease and allergy. In fact, "researchers now estimate that more than two-thirds of all immune activity occurs in the gut."[9] Allergies appear when the body develops antibodies to the (undigested) proteins derived from previously harmless food. These antibodies can enter any tissue and trigger an inflammatory reaction when that food is eaten. According to Zoltan P. Rona, M.D.:

> If this inflammation occurs in a joint, autoimmune arthritis (rheumatoid arthritis) develops. If it occurs in the brain, myalgic encephalomyelitis (a.k.a. chronic fatigue syndrome) may be the result. If it occurs in the blood vessels, vasculitis (inflammation of the blood vessels) is the resulting autoimmune problem. If the antibodies end up attacking the lining of the gut itself, the result may be colitis or Crohn's disease. If it occurs in the lungs, asthma is triggered on a delayed basis every time the individual consumes the food which triggered the production of the antibodies in the first place.[10]

Leaky gut syndrome can cause malabsorption of many important nutrients— vitamins, minerals and amino acids— due to inflammation and the presence of many potent toxins. This malabsorption can also cause gas, bloating and cramps and eventually such complaints as fatigue, headaches, memory loss, poor concentration and irritability. The set of symptoms known collectively as **irritable bowel syndrome** (IBS)—bloating and gas after eating and alternating constipation and diarrhea—has also been linked to leaky gut syndrome, as has eczema.

Because of our high stress lifestyles, many of us have an overworked, under-functioning digestive system, imbalanced intestinal flora and a continuous flow of intestinal toxins seeping into the bloodstream. Why then do some people seem unaffected, able to eat or drink just about anything they choose, showing no ill effects, while others experience discomfort and ultimately chronic disease? The difference has much to do with the functioning of the gallbladder and the detoxification ability of the liver. ✳

Notes

[1] John Matsen, N.D., *The Mysterious Cause of Illness*, Fischer Publishing Corporation, 1987, p. 25.

[2] Ibid.

[3] Doug A. Kaufmann, *The Fungus Link*, Mediatrition, 2000, p. 155.

[4] Jack Tips, N.D., Ph.D, *Conquering Candida*, Apple-A-Day Press, 1995, p. 37.

[5] Op. Cit., Kaufmann, p. 148.

[6] Trent W. Nichols, M.D. and Nancy Faass, M.S.W., M.M.P.H., *Optimal Digestion*, Quill, 1999, p. 147.

[7] Ibid., p. 148.

[8] Elizabeth Lipski, M.S., C.C.N., *Digestive Wellness*, Keats Publishing, Inc., 1996, p. 778.

[9] Wendy Marson, "Gut Reactions," *Newsweek*, November 17, 1997, p. 95–99.

[10] http://www.naturallink.com/homepages/zoltan_rona/leaky

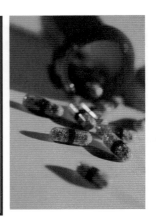

> "...inflammation in the intestinal wall (called enteritis) ...develops in 70% of people taking NSAIDs daily for two weeks."
>
> Leo Galland, MD, *The Four Pillars of Healing*

Chapter Summary

As our figure 2 flow chart indicates, impaired digestion leads to imbalanced gut flora, wherein bacteria act upon undigested food in the gut, producing endotoxins. Intestinal toxemia can lead to an overgrowth of putrefactive bacteria and often candida. Overgrowth of candida is often accompanied by parasites. Proliferation of these opportunistic organisms further upsets the bacterial balance in the intestines. An overgrowth of pathogenic bacteria and intestinal toxemia can cause irritation of the intestinal tract, tissue damage and impaired circulation, any of which can lead to gastrointestinal inflammation.

The intestinal wall cannot renew itself without sufficient beneficial flora to ferment dietary fiber into short-chain fatty acids. Leaky gut syndrome occurs when the mucosal lining of the intestinal tract becomes porous and irritated. As time passes, the breakdown in the intestinal mucosa can result in the passage of undigested food particles, toxins, parasites and candida by-products into the bloodstream. This can lead to a weakened immune system, digestive disorders and, eventually, chronic disease.

Your digestive

H igh fiber O il P robiotics E nzymes

for the future

Today's health care consumers can be completely overwhelmed with all of the good options that are available to enhance health. So, to simplify the choices, we recommend seven options that are the foundation of nutritional health. HOPE AAA:

High-fiber diet – a balance of soluble and insoluble fiber.

Oils – essential fatty acids, predominantly Omega-3, with some Omega-6 and liberal use of extra virgin cold-pressed olive oil (Omega-9).

Probiotics – several species of lactobacilli and bifidobacteria, at least 6 billion organisms per day, along with prebiotics (FOS and inulin) to support the bacteria.

Enzymes – Plant-based enzymes to be taken with meals (especially with cooked foods) to assist in digestion of protein, fat and carbohydrates. This is especially important over age 50.

Antioxidants - free radical scavengers, vitamin A, vitamin C, vitamin E, selenium, zinc, glutathione, lipoic acid, to name a few (see appendix for details).

Anti-inflammatory compounds – Many herbs like Boswellia, curcumin, silymarin, dandelion, marshmallow, slippery elm and aloe have the ability to lower inflammation in the GI tract (as well as in the entire body).

Alkaline diet – At least 80% of everyone's diet should include vegetables, fruits, seeds, nuts and sprouted grains and legumes to create an alkaline mineral reserve in the body. If the first morning urine pH is lower than 6.5, it is a general indication that the body may be too acidic. This occurs with inadequate fluid intake and excess stress, as well as with a diet high in protein, animal fats, simple carbohydrates and excess sugars and sodas.

There is tremendous synergy when all seven of the above options are combined together to promote gastrointestinal health and thereby total body health. It is interesting to note that the HOPE-AAA style of eating, which emphasizes whole, raw, fermented, sprouted and organic foods, has been the mainstay of the human diet since the beginning of recorded history. Today, however, processed, chemically preserved foods and high-yield chemical agricultural methods have become the norm. Their devitalizing effect has made nutritional supplentation a necessary fact of life.

Fiber, oils, probiotics, digestive enzymes, antioxidants, and anti-inflammatories, all of which are critical for optimum health (especially with aging), are now available and recommended dietary supplements. But most important is to choose a diet of whole organic foods whenever possible.

CHAPTER 4

H.O.P.E.
high fiber

One of the causes of overweight is the body's retention of water and fat to try to dilute pesticides and other poisons.

Source:
Surviving the Toxic Crisis
by Dr. William R. Kellas and
Dr. Andrea Sharon Dworkin.

WHAT IS IT?

The fiber component of food, known as "dietary fiber," is a type of complex carbohydrate found only in plants, primarily in their cell walls. Fiber is not technically a nutrient since we humans cannot digest it. While it contains no nutrients, the food in which fiber is found is loaded with them. For our purposes we want to concentrate on the health-associated benefits of having a high-fiber diet. A high-fiber diet, as we recommend it, includes 35 grams of fiber daily for women and up to 45 grams per day for men. This amount is hard to obtain through regular dietary consumption (the average American gets just 15-20 grams), so supplementation is usually necessary. Before we go into the specific health-related benefits of a high-fiber diet, let's first take a deeper look at fiber in its different forms, and consider the sources from which it comes.

Types and Sources
No animal products contain any fiber, nor does sugar. It's only found in plant foods like fruits, vegetables, nuts, seeds and grains. There are two basic types of fiber, soluble and insoluble, as indicated below:

Soluble and Insoluble
Soluble fiber (pectin, gum and mucilage) dissolves and breaks down in water, forming a gummy gel. Insoluble fiber (cellulose, hemicellulose and lignin), a.k.a. roughage or crude fiber, does not dissolve in water or break down at all. It passes through the gastrointestinal tract almost intact. Most plant foods contain a combination of both types of fiber in varying amounts. The chart on the page 45 shows some foods that are rich in either soluble or insoluble fiber.

It is important to consume both soluble and insoluble fiber, for each type has its unique benefits, as the chart indicates. An imbalance can create problems. Psyllium, the major type of fiber sold in health food stores and the main ingredient in a lot of commercial bulk laxatives, is

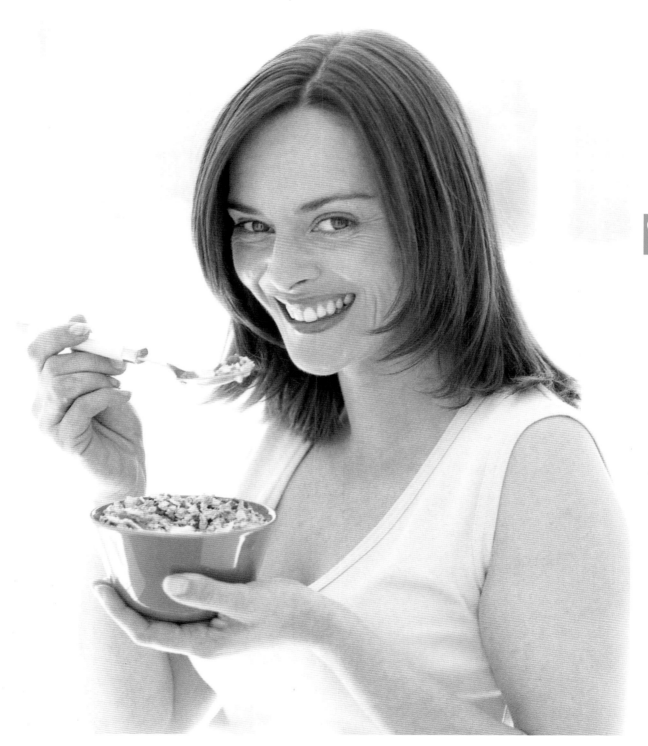

4

Fiber	
Insoluble Fiber	**Soluble Fiber**
• Brazil nuts • Brown rice • Peanuts • Popcorn • Wheat bran • Whole grain breads, cereals, pastas • Vegetables (green beans, cauliflower, potato skins, root vegetable skins) • Fruit skins • Flax seed	• Barley • Fruits (apples, citrus, cranberries, grapes, peaches, pears, prunes, sour plums) • Vegetables (beets, carrots) • Legumes (peas, lentils and dried beans) • Oats (oat bran and oatmeal) • Psyllium husks (not recommended: see next paragraph) • Rye • Seeds (including flax) • Guar gum

97% water-soluble and actually absorbs 40 times its own weight in water. The down side of this is that it has a dehydrating effect on the colon. Over-consumption of psyllium can therefore cause constipation (as well as bloating). Ironically, many people are taking fiber because they are already constipated and are unaware that it can actually make the problem worse. Two other problems associated with eating a high level of psyllium fiber, according to Leo Galland, M.D., are that it (1) can increase intestinal permeability and create changes in the internal environment that contribute to the development of stomach or bowel cancer and (2) can encourage "an overgrowth of the normal intestinal bacteria, which deprives the body of vitamin B12 and produces an increase in the concentration of bacterial toxins."[1]

Dietary Fiber
Fiber works by two different mechanisms: Soluble fiber acts like a sponge, actually absorbing toxins

as it passes through the gastrointestinal tract. It also slows down the absorption of nutrients. This can work to our advantage if we are trying to lose weight. By slowing down glucose absorption, blood sugar levels are kept balanced, which will keep your appetite in check and stave off sugar cravings.

Because insoluble fiber (also known as "roughage") does not break down, it will sweep clean the GI tract, scrubbing off toxins in the bowel as it encounters them. Insoluble fiber also tones the bowel by creating resistance, giving the muscles of the colon some exercise by providing something for them to push against. This increases peristalsis, the muscle motion necessary for good

Health Benefits of Soluble and Insoluble Fiber

Insoluble Fiber
• Is good for hemorrhoids, varicose veins, and colitis.
• Is good for promoting weight loss, relieving constipation, preventing colon cancer and controlling carcinogens in the intestinal tract.
• Is good for lowering cholesterol levels. It helps to prevent the formation of gallstones by binding with bile acids and removing cholesterol before stones can form. It is beneficial for persons with diabetes.

Soluble Fiber
• Helps regulate blood sugar levels, lower cholesterol and remove toxins.
• Slows the absorption of food after meals and is therefore good for people with diabetes. It also removes unwanted metals and toxins, reduces the side effects of radiation therapy, helps lower cholesterol and reduces the risk of heart disease and gallstones.

From *Prescription for Nutritional Healing* by Phyllis A. Balch, C.N.C., and James F. Balch, M.D., pgs. 69-70

elimination. A blend of both soluble and insoluble dietary fiber will bind toxins and increase elimination without the undesirable side effects of a single fiber such as psyllium.

Constipation

As mentioned, eating dietary fiber is the best way to get and stay regular. Long-term chronic constipation is usually caused by two factors: dehydration and insufficient dietary fiber. The muscles of the colon, just like any other muscles, need to be exercised in order to stay "fit." Dietary fiber in the digestive tract creates bulk or matter for these muscles to work and push against, keeping them strong and healthy. The typical American diet contains about 15-20 grams of dietary fiber per day. This is low even by conservative standards. Some people eat even less than this. Years of consuming low dietary fiber cause the muscles of the colon to become weak and atrophied. When this happens, chronic constipation can be the result. This is often compounded by the fact that people do not drink enough water. The colon is a recycling center for water; 80% of the water is extracted out of fecal material as it passes through the colon. When a person does not drink enough water to properly hydrate the bowel, constipation can result.

Heart Disease/Cholesterol

Cholesterol is both produced and processed for elimination in the liver. The liver produces aproximately 85% of your body's total cholesterol. Cholesterol, which is a fatty substance, cannot be eliminated by the body in its fat-soluble (dissolves in fat) state. After it has served its purpose, it is sent back to the liver to be converted into a form that can be eliminated by the body. The liver uses a complex chemical process to change the cholesterol from a fat-soluble to a water-soluble substance. Once this occurs, the water-soluble cholesterol is put into bile, which is also produced by the liver. This bile is then sent to the gallbladder for storage and later use. Part of the function of bile is to help in the digestion (emulsification) of fats. Bile is

also a vehicle to move toxins out of the body. The components of bile are bile salts and toxins (used up cholesterol, histamine, hormones, dead red blood cells etc.) When fat is eaten, the gallbladder is stimulated to release small amounts of bile into the digestive tract. This bile, along with all of its components, including cholesterol, are bound up in fiber and carried out of the body in a bowel movement. In a person who eats insufficient fiber, the toxins have nothing to bind to and end up being reabsorbed through the blood vessels that line the colon in the water reabsorption process. These toxins end up in the liver once again and stagnate and overburden the liver. In this manner, insufficient dietary fiber can lead to a blood test that reflects not only today's cholesterol in the blood, but also yesterday's and cholesterol from the days before. A high-fiber diet will have the effect of absorbing the water-soluble cholesterol, thus reducing blood cholesterol levels.

Diabetes/Blood Sugar Regulation

When carbohydrate foods are eaten in their natural (unprocessed/high-fiber) state, the sugars that they contain are bound up in dietary fiber, making it harder for the body to get at them. This slows their breakdown and subsequent absorption and has the effect of making their entry into the bloodstream more gradual and consistent. This will have the effect of regulating blood sugar levels.

We now have a better idea of what fiber is and what it does. Now let's take a look at some foods and their fiber content.

High-Fiber Foods

The following list (p. 49) represents the total fiber content of foods per serving. Serving size is based on a 2000-calorie per day diet. All fruits and vegetables are raw unless otherwise noted. Please note: Measurements can be confusing when it comes to food products. Food can be measured by capacity (volume), or by weight. Eight ounces is not necessarily equivalent to eight fluid ounces or one cup. Eight ounces is a measure of how much something weighs; one cup is a measure of how much space it occupies. For instance, a cup of popcorn weighs about one ounce, but eight ounces of popcorn would fill many cups. For the purpose of this list, you are comparing apples to apples, as they say. All amounts compare serving sizes based on the same amount of food. Also consider that these foods are listed raw. When you cook vegetables, they become pliable and much more of them fit into the same space, which raises fiber content for the same volume.

Although there is no food group better for you than fruits and vegetables, many people have misconceptions about the volume of food intake required to meet suggested healthy dietary fiber levels. For instance many people who eat a salad for lunch would tell you so as a testament to their good health practices, weight loss and/or maintenance strategy or desire to eat more fiber. Did you know that an average salad, even a big one, contains no more than 2 grams of fiber? In other words, to meet the dietary fiber intake recommended by the FDA of 25 grams per day (which is low by our standards), you'd have to eat 12½ salads per day. We have compiled the following information in the hopes that you will use it to make healthier food choices. Since some fruits and vegetables are much higher than others in fiber content, it would be wise to start substituting those with higher

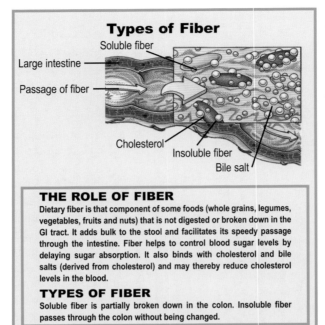

Types of Fiber

Soluble fiber

Large intestine

Passage of fiber

Cholesterol

Insoluble fiber

Bile salt

THE ROLE OF FIBER

Dietary fiber is that component of some foods (whole grains, legumes, vegetables, fruits and nuts) that is not digested or broken down in the GI tract. It adds bulk to the stool and facilitates its speedy passage through the intestine. Fiber helps to control blood sugar levels by delaying sugar absorption. It also binds with cholesterol and bile salts (derived from cholesterol) and may thereby reduce cholesterol levels in the blood.

TYPES OF FIBER

Soluble fiber is partially broken down in the colon. Insoluble fiber passes through the colon without being changed.

amounts for those that are lower in fiber. The list goes from foods of highest fiber content to lowest fiber content by category, so if you currently eat the ones at the bottom, start eating the ones at the top!!! Knowledge is power.

Where food labeling is concerned, in order for a packaged food product to be called "high-fiber," one serving must contain 5 grams of fiber or more. For it to be called a "good source of fiber," it must contain between 2.5 and 4.9 grams. According to this information, many fruits and vegetables fall below even "good" levels of dietary fiber. This is not to say, "don't eat them." We encourage you to eat as much as you can as often as you can. What we are saying is that it is much easier to reach the level of fiber intake that we suggest if you eat well and also supplement.

Legumes, like most grains, contain substances named phytates, which are called and considered "antinutrients." Phytates bind to, and therefore block, the absorption of vitamins and minerals like iron, magnesium, vitamin B and calcium. It is for this reason that we do not recommend legumes and grains as the staple of your diet. Legumes and grains do contain high amounts of fiber, and so if you do eat them, eat them moderately. Beans and grains should always be soaked overnight, as this removes most of the phytates.

Notes

[1] Leo Galland, M.D., *The Four Pillars of Healing*, Random House, 1997, p. 196.

VEGETABLES

Vegetable / Amount	Total Fiber
Acorn squash, 1/2 cup cooked	4.5 grams
Sauerkraut, 1/2 cup	4 grams
Sweet potato, 1 medium	3.5 grams
Potato, 1 medium	3 grams
Corn, 1/2 cup off cob	3 grams
Beets, 1 medium	2.5 grams
Broccoli, 1/2 cup	2 grams
Brussell sprouts, 1/2 cup	2 grams
Carrots, 1/2 cup	2 grams
Cauliflower, 1/2 cup	2 grams
Eggplant, 1/2 cup	2 grams
Rutabaga, 1/2 cup	2 grams
Spinach, 1/2 cup	2 grams
Turnip greens, 1/2 cup	2 grams
Collard greens, 1/2 cup	1.5 grams
Crook neck squash, 1/2 cup	1.5 grams
Mustard greens, 1/2 cup	1.5 grams
Cabbage, 1/2 cup	1 gram
Celery, 1/2 cup	1 gram
Kale, 1/2 cup	1 gram
Leek, 1/2 cup	1 gram
Popcorn, 1 cup popped	1 gram
Zucchini, 1/2 cup	1 gram
Lettuce, 1/2 cup	.5 gram
All pre-cut packaged lettuce mixes, 1/2 cup	.5 gram

GRAINS

Grain / Amount	Total Fiber
Amaranth, 1 oz.	4.3 grams
Barley, 1 oz.	3 grams
Teff, 1 oz.	4 grams
Spelt, 1 oz.	4 grams
Rye, 1 oz.	3 grams
Wheat, 1 oz.	3 grams
Oats, 1 oz.	3 grams
Millet, 1 oz.	2.5 grams
Bulgur, 1 oz.	2 grams
Kamut, 1 oz.	2 grams
Quinoa, 1 oz.	1.5 grams

FRUITS

Fruit / Amount	Total Fiber
Coconut, 1/2 cup	8 grams
Orange, 1 medium	7 grams
Grapefruit, 1/2 large	6 grams
Raisins, 1/2 cup	6 grams
Dates, 1/2 cup	6 grams
Kiwi, 2 medium	5.2 grams
Apple, 1 medium	5 grams
Blackberries, 1/2 cup	5 grams
Persimmons, 1 medium	5 grams
Elderberries, 1/2 cup	5 grams
Honeydew melon, 1/2 melon	5 grams
Banana, 1 medium	4 grams
Papaya, 1/2 large	4 grams
Pear, 1 medium	4 grams
Raspberries, 1/2 cup	4 grams
Cantaloupe, 1 medium	4 grams
Carambola (star fruit), 1 medium	3.5 grams
Currants, 1/2 cup	3 grams
Tangerine, 1 medium	3 grams
Apricot, 3 medium	2.5 grams
Blueberries, 1/2 cup	2 grams
Cranberries, 1/2 cup	2 grams
Mango, 1 medium	2 grams
Nectarine, 1 medium	2 grams
Peach, 1 medium	2 grams
Plum, 2 medium	2 grams
Strawberries, 1/2 cup	2 grams
Tomato, 1 medium	2 grams
Cherries, 1/2 cup	1.5 grams
Pineapple, 1/2 cup	1 gram
Grapes, 1/2 cup	< 1 gram

LEGUMES (BEANS)

Legumes / Amount	Total Fiber
Red beans, 1/2 cup	9 grams
Adzuki, 1/2 cup	8.5 grams
Lentil, 1/2 cup	8 grams
Crowder peas, 1/2 cup	8 grams
Mung, 1/2 cup	7.7 grams
Black, 1/2 cup	7.5 grams
Pinto, 1/2 cup	7.3 grams
Chili, 1/2 cup	7 grams
Garbanzo (chick peas), 1/2 cup	7 grams
Great northern, 1/2 cup	7 grams
Kidney, 1/2 cup	7 Grams
Lima, 1/2 cup	7 grams
Navy, 1/2 cup	6 grams
Anasazi, 1/2 cup	4.5 grams
Appaloosa, 1/2 cup	4.5 grams
Field peas, 1/2 cup	4 grams
Green peas, 1/2 cup	4 grams
Edamame (soy), 1/2 cup	3.8 grams
Green beans, 1/2 cup	2 grams

4

H.O.P.E.
HIGH FIBER
SUPPLEMENT RECOMMENDATIONS

As you can see, you'd have to eat a tremendous amount of fruits and vegetables to attain the recommended 35-45 grams of fiber daily. It is for this reason we recommend that in addition to eating a healthy and balanced high-fiber diet, you also take a fiber supplement. We recommend a fiber supplement that has a blend of the two types of dietary fiber (soluble and insoluble) that your body needs. Flax, acacia and oat bran make a good blend of fiber. This blend will ensure that you receive all of the health associated benefits of fiber.

CHAPTER 5

H.O.P.E.
oils ESSENTIAL FATTY ACIDS

Happiness is nothing more than good health and bad memory.

Source:
Albert Schweitzer

In today's fat-conscious climate, fats in general have gotten a bad rap. While there are some fats that can be harmful to your health, they are not the ones that most people think they are, and the information of the last 20 years is confusing to the consumer at best. Research into "what is the right fat" is conflicting. First we were told that margarine is better for us than butter. Some scientists then did a complete turn-around to say butter should be eaten instead of margarine. We were told that eggs raised our cholesterol levels, only to be told 10 years later that they had little effect and in fact were good to eat in moderation. This chapter will unravel some of this information and leave you with a clear sense of what fats are good to eat and use as a dietary supplement.

SATURATED FATS

Saturated fats are semi-solid at room temperature and are found in animal products such as red meat, lamb and pork, and in dairy products such as cheese, butter and milk. Saturated fats are also found in processed foods. They are generally considered "bad fats," as they can contribute to heart disease, so it is generally recommended to eat these in moderation.

Not all saturated fats are the same. There are three subgroups based on the length of their fat chain: short, medium and long.

Good
Short-chain saturates such as those found in butter, coconut oil and palm oil, do not clog arteries or cause heart disease. They are easily digested and are a source of fuel for immediate energy.

The Not Too Bad
Medium-chain saturates are found in many foods, but the highest content is also found in palm and coconut oils. They are not shown to increase cholesterol or risk of heart disease.

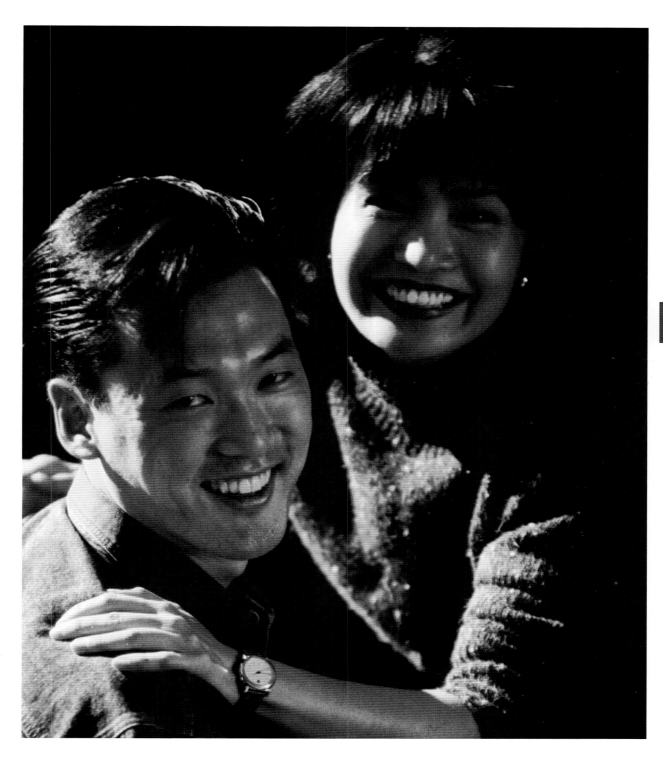

Bad

Long-chain saturates are the fats associated with raising LDL (bad cholesterol) while lowering HDL (good cholesterol) and therefore increasing the risk of heart disease. The bad fats are those found in meat. Long-chain saturates are also the by-product of hydrogenation, which means they are found in margarine, shortening, restaurant fried foods and most anything that comes in a box or off of a grocery store shelf.

Unsaturated Fats

Unsaturated fats are liquid at room temperature and are considered to be the good fats. These fats are subcategorized as monounsaturated or polyunsaturated. Monounsaturated fats remain liquid at room temperature but solidify in colder temperatures. These include olive, canola and peanut oil (more about canola oil in chapter 8). Polyunsaturated fats remain liquid even in cold temperatures and include flax, borage, corn, safflower, sesame, soy, sunflower, evening primrose oils and fatty fish.

Supplemental EFAs

Some fatty acids (the main components of all fats) actually help produce hormones and a multitude of other substances in the body. These fatty acids are known as essential fatty acids (EFAs). They are "good fats," the omega-3 and omega-6 fatty acids. They are called "essential" because they are essential to life, and your body can't manufacture them. They must be obtained through food and/or through dietary supplements.

In addition to their role in hormone production, EFAs do the following:

- Are used to manufacture the cell wall of every cell in the body
- Support the cardiovascular, reproductive, immune and nervous systems
- Increase the absorption of vitamins and minerals

- Lubricate the colon
- Promote proper nerve functioning
- Help support gastrointestinal health
- Relieve inflammatory conditions

Signs and symptoms of essential fatty acid deficiency:

- Dry, scaly skin or other skin problems
- Fatigue
- Impaired growth and fertility
- Losses in visual acuity
- Neuropathies (nervous system disorders)
- Organ damage and failure

The bottom line is that EFAs are required for the proper structure and function of every cell in the body, and Americans are not getting enough of them. An estimated 80% of us are deficient in the EFAs, particularly omega-3s (found primarily in cold water fish and flax seeds). There are many reasons for this deficiency, including:

- Removal of EFA-containing germ from flour when it is milled
- Consumption of sugar and fried foods that may interfere with EFA absorption
- Decreased consumption of fish
- Increased intake of "trans fats" (hydrogenated oils) found in processed foods which may interfere with absorption of EFAs
- Increased use of refined oils that do not contain EFAs
- Adherence to a fat-free or reduced-fat diet

Flax seeds contain both types of EFAs but a larger percentage of omega-3. Omega-6 EFAs are primarily found in animal products and commonly used cooking oils. Because Americans typically consume large quantities of these, the balance between omega-3s and omega-6s has been tipped in favor of omega-6s. Eating more omega-3-rich fats from fish, vegetables, flax seed oil and walnuts, as well as using appropriate omega-3 supplements, can help restore this balance.

When supplementing, look for an omega-3 formula, from fish that contains a concentrated ratio of 300mg EPA to 200 mg DH4 per capsule. To assure proper fat digestion, you'll want to select an omega-3 formula that contains the fat-digesting enzyme lipase. Look for enteric coated dark gel caps (that help prevent oxidation of the oil), and take a minimum of 1 to 3 per day, with or following meals. You may also want to use liquid flax oil as a salad dressing. Never cook with it, however, as it is extremely heat-sensitive.

Oils in the Diet

All oils have some degree of heat sensitivity. They are also sensitive to light and air. Exposure to heat, light and/or oxygen results in oxidation, or rancidity, in oils. For this reason, most oils should be refrigerated. Good oil kept under improper conditions can easily become bad for you. An exception is coconut oil, which can be safely stored at room temperature. This oil, due to its ability to withstand high temperatures, is ideal to use for baking or frying, where intense heat is applied. In addition to cooking with it, you may wish to add coconut oil to smoothies to enhance their flavor and nutritional value.

While coconut oil is a versatile and healthy choice, there are also other healthy options. Olive oil (choose virgin olive oil) is a good choice for sautéing. It may also be used for stir-frying; butter is also a good choice for most cooking purposes.

Bad Oils

It is advisable to avoid margarine and vegetable shortenings, as these contain harmful trans fats. Trans fats, found in hydrogenated or partially hydrogenated oils, are lacking in natural fat emulsifiers. They inhibit gallbladder function and damage the liver. Hydrogenated fats also promote inflammation, inhibit the absorption of fat-soluble vitamins by binding with them in your body, raise LDL ("bad cholesterol") levels and lead to clogged

arteries, diabetes and more. By avoiding processed foods, you will be minimizing your exposure to harmful trans fats.

The trans fats, not animal fats, are your major "bad fats." Any refined oil would also fall in this category. Refined oils are not labeled as such. If the oil is light and crystal clear, it is probably refined. Such oils constitute the bulk of those found on supermarket shelves. The refining process removes important nutrients from these oils, including the fat emulsifier lecithin and the fat-digesting enzyme lipase. Fat utilization becomes problematic in the face of deficiencies of these important nutrients. This, in turn, presents an obstacle to your efforts to maintain or regain your health.

To avoid the hazards posed by refined oils, you'll want to select only unrefined oils. These are generally found in health food stores or in the "natural foods" or "specialty foods" section of your supermarket. These oils may be labeled as "unrefined," or they may be labeled as "cold-pressed," "cold-processed," or "expeller-pressed." In addition, you'll want to opt for organic oils whenever possible.

As you can see, fats are necessary to live a long, healthy life. Like all things, it is a matter of finding the proper balance. Once you have found the balance that is right for you, there will be visible changes in your appearance (hair, skin and nails) and also changes at the cellular level that you may not see but should definitely feel.

H.O.P.E.
Oil
SUPPLEMENT RECOMMENDATIONS

We recommend taking 2 grams per day of omega-3 oils. Look for a formulation that also contains lipase, is enteric coated and comes in dark gel caps to filter out light.

CHAPTER 6

H.O.P.E.

probiotics
GOOD BACTERIA

A man too busy to take care of his health is like a mechanic too busy to take care of his tools.

Source:
Spanish proverb

BALANCING GUT FLORA

The intestinal tract contains more than 500 species of bacteria. It is critical to good health and the immune system that the right ratio of good bacteria to bad bacteria (80%:20%) be maintained in the intestine. If the bad, or in some cases even benign microorganisms (yeast) are prevalent, a condition called dysbiosis can occur. There are many causes of dysbiosis. It is usually self-induced, meaning it results from high levels of stress, chemical exposure, poor diet, overuse of antibiotics, birth control pills and/or drugs of all kinds. The over-prescribing of antibiotics is probably the single most responsible factor for imbalance in the digestive tract. There are ways to balance the gut flora with advanced cleansing methods. In order to establish bacterial balance, one will need to:

• Reduce bad bacteria.
• Reestablish good bacteria.

Replace Gut Flora

In order to balance gut flora, we must return the good bacteria to the digestive tract with a probiotic formula.

The term "probiotics" comes from the Greek words "pro" and "biotics," meaning "for life" or "in favor of life" respectively. Holistic practitioners often begin any discussion of probiotics with this very basic definition because of its simplicity and clarity. Probiotics are beneficial and even necessary to life. They are predominately bacterial; however, some fungi (like *Saccharomyces boulardii*) are also considered beneficial "probiotic" microorganisms.

Resident vs. Transient Strains

Another important point about beneficial bacteria involves the

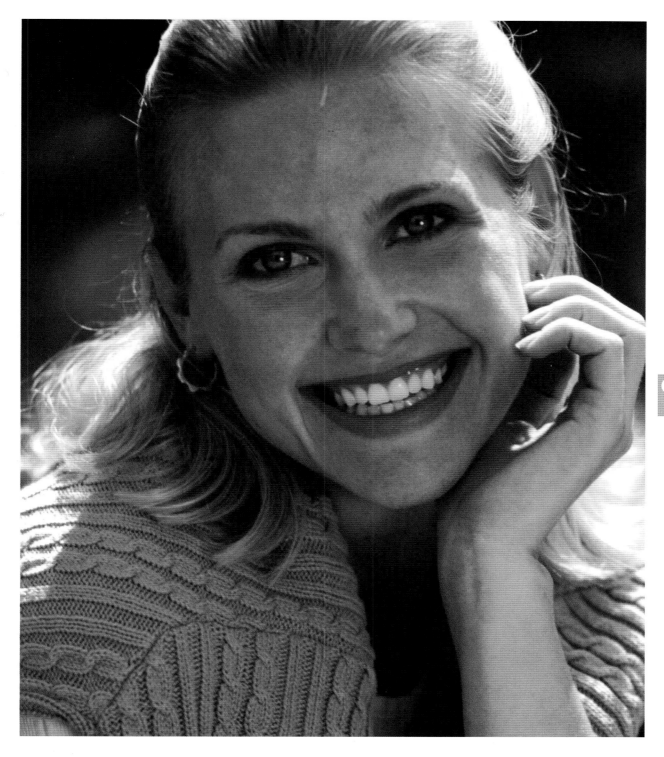

relationship between resident and transient strains. Resident strains are those strains that are commonly found in the human digestive tract. *Lactobacillus acidophilus* and *Bifidobacterium bifidum* are common resident strains found virtually in all human intestinal systems. *Lactobacillus casei, Lactobacillus bulgarius* and *Streptococcus thermophillus* are common transient strains. Transient strains are often consumed in foods like yogurt. These strains will not reestablish in the digestive tract; however, they do provide many benefits as they pass through.

Probiotics and Prebiotics

Probiotics have been defined as living micro-organisms that positively improve health and intestinal environment. A prebiotic is defined as "a non-digestible food ingredient that beneficially affects the host by selectively stimulating the growth and/or activity of one or a limited number of bacteria in the colon" (Gibson and Roberfroid, 1995). A prebiotic is further defined as a dietary ingredient that reaches the large intestine in an intact form and has a specific metabolism therein, one directed toward beneficial rather than harmful bacteria. A true prebiotic must:

1. be neither hydrolyzed nor absorbed by the upper part of the digestive tract
2. be a selective substrate (surface on which an organism can grow) for one or a limited number of beneficial bacteria
3. be able to alter the colonic flora in favor of a healthier composition
4. induce luminal (inner surface of a tubular organ) or systemic effects that are beneficial to the host

Selecting The Probiotic

There are at least 100 companies distributing probiotic products today. It is interesting to note that there are far fewer companies (perhaps a

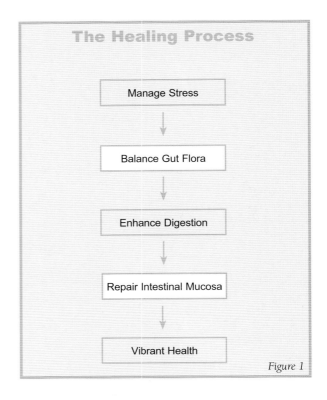

The Healing Process

Manage Stress

↓

Balance Gut Flora

↓

Enhance Digestion

↓

Repair Intestinal Mucosa

↓

Vibrant Health

Figure 1

dozen or so) that actually manufacture or culture the majority of the probiotics sold in the U.S. Companies (many of them quite large) contract with these manufacturers to produce a specific proprietary formulation that serves the particular market they are attempting to support. Each probiotic formula will be different. The products will have different types and numbers of cultures; they may or may not be packaged with a prebiotic, and they will have a broad range of prices. In order to make a selection, consider the following:

Species selection – The majority of studies have been conducted using species from either the *Lactobacillus* or *Bifidobacterium* family. These are the most prevalent beneficial genera. Since these genera have no known pathogenic species or strains, they are generally thought of as being the safest and most well-researched probiotics.

Transient vs. resident – Most probiotic

Pro, Pre and Synbiotics

PROBIOTIC

Definition	A live microbial food supplement which beneficially affects the host animal by improving its intestinal microbial balance.
Examples	lactobacilli, bifidobacteria, enterococci, streptococci
Advantages	Strain may have proven health values. Useful when gut flora may be compromised
Possible Future Developments	New product developments based on synbiotics that may improve probiotic survival

PREBIOTIC

Definition	A non-digestible food ingredient that beneficially affects the host by selectively stimulating the growth and/or activity of one or a limited number of bacteria in the colon, and thus improves host health
Examples	Frutooligosaccharides (FOS), inulin, galactooligosaccharides
Advantages	Genus-level changes occur in gut flora. Product survival not problematic. Low dose required and can be incorporated into many different food delivery systems.
Possible Future Developments	Manufacture of novel mutiple-function prebiotics, that may: stimulate the "beneficial" flora; exert anti-adhesive properties; attenuate pathogen virulence. Prebiotics derived from dietary fiber-type polysacchrides

SYNBIOTIC

Definition	A mixture of pro and prebiotics which beneficially affects the host by improving the survival and implantation of live microbial dietary supplements in the gastrointestinal tract
Examples	Frutooligosaccharides (FOS), + bifidobacteria; lactitol + lactobacilli
Advantages	Dual effect of entities. Probiotic survival should be improved.
Possible Future Developments	Design of new synbiotics through molecular engineering (based on specific prebiotic enzymes)

Chart taken from *The Advanced Guide to Longevity Medicine* by Mitchell J. Ghen, p. 213

Figure 2

6

products consist of multiple species from either the *Lactobacillus* or *Bifidobacterium* family. Some of the *Lactobacillus* species are transient bacteria (*L. casei*), and others are resident. While both resident and transient species are beneficial, resident species may offer the advantage of reestablishment in the digestive tract. Resident species may also be more likely to work together and be less antagonistic to other resident strains already in the digestive tract. One strategy is to use a product that has multiple strains of resident lactobacilli and bifidobacteria species to rebuild

and maintain the intestinal environment. Specific, well-tested transient strains (*L. casei* or *L. bulgaricus*) are then used individually to boost the maintenance dose.

Site Utilization – Species selection is also dependent on the area of the intestinal tract being targeted. Since it is often difficult to determine the specific intestinal area of need, a multi-species product that contains both lactobacillis and bifidobacteria may be the best choice because these species target both the small and large intestine.

Culture counts – Probiotics are usually measured in numbers of organisms per capsule, per tablet or per gram (in the case of powders). High-potency products typically contain 6-50 billion organisms in a capsule or tablet and four billion cultures per gram in the powder. All products should list an expiration date on the label, which would indicate how long the product will retain its stated potency.

Storage – Most of the common probiotic species, *Lactobacillus acidophilus* and *Bifidobacterium bifidum*, for example, do not survive for long periods at or above room temperatures. A few probiotics, like *Streptococcus faecium*, can survive at room temperatures. Unrefrigerated organisms do not die immediately, but if probiotics that require refrigeration are stored on the shelf for months, or beyond expiration date, the loss of potency can be significant. Even non-refrigerated species may retain potency longer in refrigeration.

Resident Strains in Humans

Lactobacillus acidophilus
Lactobacillus salivarius
Bifidobacterium bifidum
Bifidobacterium infantis
Bifidobacterium longum
Streptococcus faecalis
Streptococcus faecium

Transient Strains

Lactobacillus brevis
Lactobacillus bulgaricus
Lactobacillus casei
Lactobacillus delbrueckii
Lactobacillus kefir
Lactobacillus plantarum
Lactobacillus yoghurti
Streptococcus lactis
Streptococcus thermophilus

Figure 3

Prebiotics – There is significant research that supports the use of prebiotics in promoting enhanced levels of beneficial bacteria. Fructooligosaccharides (FOS) are added to many probiotic formulations. Prebiotics like FOS have been shown clinically to enhance the intestinal levels of beneficial probiotics. Selecting a formulation that contains multiple resident probiotics (lactobacilli, bifidobacteria) and prebiotics (FOS) is desirable.

Dosing The Probiotic

There are two considerations in selecting the ideal dose of probiotics: The first is when to take the probiotic (with meals or between meals), and the second is how much to take.

Some practitioners suggest that taking probiotics with meals can aid in digestion. Others suggest that taking probiotics between meals, when stomach acid is lowest, is best. In general, probiotics taken once or twice daily with a large glass of water, between meals can help deliver the probiotic to the intestinal tract faster and in higher concentrations.

Choosing a probiotic with a "delivery system" can take away the guesswork on when to take it. A delivery system is simply some mechanism employed to assure that a sufficient number of live organisms will survive the hydrochloric acid (HCl) of the stomach and make it through to the colon. If your probiotic has an efficient delivery system, it will do its job virtually any time you take it.

One effective delivery system is the patented Bio-tract™ technology, which utilizes a protective gel layer that protects the probiotics through the stomach acid, once the tablet is hydrated. This technology allows the safe delivery of at least 80% of the tablet's weight to the intestine, where the probiotics are needed. Because of the protective gel layer, which protects the friendly bacteria from stomach acid, the tablet can be taken any time of day without regard to elevated HCl from meals. Look for a probiotic that will safely deliver 6 billion cultures employing the Bio-tract™ delivery technology.

An alternative way of assuring that your probiotic will survive the acidic environment of the stomach is to select an enteric-coated vegetable capsule. An enteric coating is a water-based coating that helps protect the living probiotic cultures from HCl. 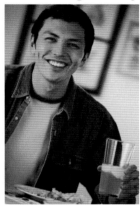 Your level of health will determine the appropriate potency. If you are taking the probiotic strictly for maintenance, a product containing 5 to 15 billion cultures is fine. If you have gastro-intestinal health issues, you will want to look for one that contains 50 billion cultures.

Research continues to support the holistic concept that achieving long-term vibrant health is dependant on having balanced body systems that function together. The digestive system is one of the most important, and in some ways least understood, of these systems. A balanced intestinal environment is a critical component of any healthy digestive system. Practitioners today have a variety of new tools to use that can help them help their patients achieve improved digestive health. Probiotics, prebiotics, enzymes and amino compounds can be used to help maintain a healthy intestinal eco-system and extended longevity.

Some Beneficial Microflora and their Characteristics

Lactobacillus acidophilus – is a natural bacteria that inhabits the small and large intestines of humans and animals. Facultative anaerobic lacto-bacilli (meaning they can grow in the absence as well as the presence of oxygen) produce lactic acid as a main product from carbohydrates. Their optimum growth temperature is 95°-100°F. The major beneficial functions of acido-bacteria are:

1. They enhance and allow digestion of milk sugar (lactose) by producing the enzyme lactase, and generally aid in the digestion of nutrients
2. They are capable by some competitive means, by the creation of lactic acid and by other inhibitory substances, of suppressing undesirable microorganisms in the intestines
3. Some strains help to destroy hostile invading bacteria by producing natural antibiotic substances
4. Some strains help to reduce the level of cholesterol, thus lessening the dangers of cardiovascular complications
5. They help to lessen the proliferation of hostile yeast such as *Candida albicans*

When the intestinal microflora are disturbed (the lactobacilli adversely affected) under the influence of oral antibiotic therapy, or stress conditions, the use of supplemental acidophilus, in food or concentrated form, can help reverse such negative processes. The regular use of acidophilus bacteria, as a supplement or in food, is a protective measure against an imbalance of the intestinal microflora.

Bifidobacterium bifidum – is a natural inhabitant of the human intestines but also found in the human vagina. B. bifidum occurs in larger numbers in the large intestine than in the lower part of the small intestine. They and other bifidobacteria species are the predominant organisms in the large intestine of breast-fed infants, accounting for approximately 99% of the microflora. In adolescents and adults, bifidobacteria are a major component of the large intestine's microflora. The level of bifidobacteria declines with age and also in various conditions of ill-health. They produce acetic

6

and lactic acid, with small amounts of formic acid from fermentable carbohydrates. They are anaerobic bacteria with an optimum growth temperature of 98°-105°F. The major beneficial functions are:

1. The prevention of the colonization of the intestine by invading pathogenic bacteria or yeast with which they compete for nutrients and attachment sites

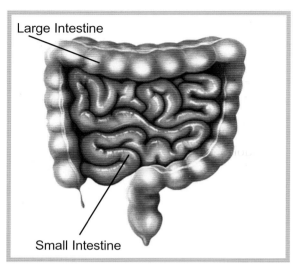
Large Intestine

Small Intestine

2. The production of acetic and lactic acids that lower the pH of the intestines, thus making the region undesirable for other possibly harmful bacteria
3. Assistance in nitrogen retention and weight gain in infants
4. The inhibition of bacteria that can alter nitrates in the intestines (derived from food or water) into potentially harmful nitrites
5. The production of B vitamins
6. Assistance in the dietary management of liver conditions

When the intestinal microflora are disturbed—and consequently Bifidobacteria decline—under the influence of oral antibiotic therapy, therapeutic irradiation of the abdomen, reduced gastric acidity, impaired intestinal motility, stresses or some other conditions, bifidobacteria supplements or bifidobacteria found in food products, such as bifidus milk, can help to restore the intestinal microflora.)

Lactobacillus salivarius – bacteria are natural residents of the human intestine and mouth. These are facultative anaerobic lacobacilli that produce lactic acid as a main product from carbohydrates. Their optimum growth temperature is 95°-104°F. As with other lactic acid bacteria, they encourage,

because of their creation of lactic acid, a more acidic environment in which less desirable microorganisms are inhibited.

Bifidobacterium infantis – is a natural inhabitant of the intestines of human infants, but also occurs in small numbers in the human vagina. Together with other bifidobacteria species, such as *B. bifidum* and *B. longum*, they are the predominant organisms in the large intestine of infants. They are anaerobic bacteria that produce acetic and lactic acids and small amounts of formic acid from carbohydrates. The major beneficial functions are similar to those of *B. bifidum*:

1. The prevention of the colonization of the intestine by invading pathogenic bacteria or yeast with which they compete for nutrients and attachments sites
2. The production of acetic and lactic acids that lower the pH of the intestine, thus making the region undesirable for other possibly harmful bacteria
3. Assistance in nitrogen retention and weight gain in infants
4. The inhibition of bacteria, which can alter nitrates into potentially harmful nitrites
5. The production of B vitamins

When the intestinal microflora of infants is disturbed (and the levels of bifidobacteria decline) under the influence of sudden changes in nutrition, use of antibiotics, vaccinations, convalescences or sudden weather changes, the use of bifidobacteria supplements or bifidobacteria found in food products can help in the nutritional restoration of the intestinal microflora.

Bifidobacterium longum – is a natural inhabitant of the human intestine. B. longum bacteria are found in the stools of human infants and adults. Together with other bifidobacteria species, such as B. *bifidum* and B. *longum*, they are the predominant bacteria in the large intestine of infants. A separate biotype—a genetic variation within a species of B. *longum* occurs in large numbers in the large intestine of adolescents and adults. They are anaerobic bacteria that produce acetic and lactic acids with small amounts of formic acid from carbohydrates. They ferment a wider range of carbohydrates compared with B. *bifidum*. The beneficial roles are similar to those of B. *bifidum*:

1. The prevention of the colonization of the intestine by invading pathogenic bacteria or yeast with which they compete for nutrients and attachment sites
2. The production of organic acids that increase the acidity of the intestine and thereby inhibit undesirable bacteria
3. Assistance in nitrogen retention and weight gain in infants
4. The inhibition of bacteria, which can alter nitrates into potentially harmful nitrites
5. The production of B vitamins

If the intestinal micro-flora are disturbed (and the levels of bifidobacteria decline) under the influence of antibiotics, irradiation of the abdomen with gamma or x-rays, reduced gastric acidity or stress conditions, the use of bifidobacteria supplements or bifidobacteria found in food products can help in the nutritional restoration of the intestinal microflora.

A good probiotic formula should contain the resident strains of *Lactobacillus acidophilus*, *Bifidobacterium bifidum* and *Bifidobacterium infantis*. Once the bad bacteria are killed, good bacteria must replace them. This is accomplished with a probiotic supplement, preferably one with about

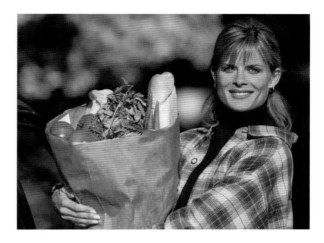

5 to 15 billion cultures per capsule. Probiotics should be taken in supplement form during the healing process and after antibiotics.

Cultured Vegetables

In addition to probiotic supplements, another good source of friendly bacteria is raw cultured vegetables. These nutrient-dense fermented foods have been around for centuries. They are rich in lactobacilli and enzymes, are alkaline-forming, an excellent source of vitamin C, an effective digestive aid, ideal for pregnant and nursing women, effective in promoting longevity and ideal for appetite control and weight control, as they reduce the cravings for sweets.

Cultured vegetables are "sauerkraut" (sauer = sour and kraut = greens or plants), not to be confused with the salted, pasteurized variety of sauerkraut sold in supermarkets. The appendix has instructions on how to make cultured vegetables.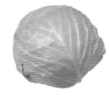

Yogurt and kefir (a creamy drink made of fermented cow's milk) are excellent sources of beneficial bacteria. The Resource Directory lists sources of high-quality kefir products.

Nutrient Support

Many people believe they can get all the nutrients they need from a "balanced diet." Others believe vitamin and mineral supplement are necessary. There's truth to both sides of this issue. Today's produce is seriously lacking in minerals. Consider this quote from U.S. Senate Document #265:

The alarming fact is that food—fruits and vegetables and grains—now being raised on millions of acres of land that no longer contains enough of needed minerals—are starving us no matter how much of them we eat. No man of today can eat enough fruits and vegetables to supply his system with the mineral salts he requires for perfect health because his stomach isn't big enough to hold them...

This document was written in 1936! The situation is even worse today as far as soil erosion is concerned. Between 1950 and 1975, the calcium content in a cup of rice decreased 21%, iron content fell 28.6%, and protein content likewise declined. As nutrients continue to be depleted in the soil, nutritional deficiencies are now the norm, even if the average person makes wise food selections and tries to eat a balanced diet. That would seem to make a case for vitamin and mineral supplements. While these may be of some benefit, whole foods are preferred, as they have a broader spectrum of nutrients in them, and their nutrients are more usable by the body than isolated ones found in vitamin and mineral pills. Whole foods contain more than just vitamins and minerals: all the nutrients contained in them haven't even been discovered, much less duplicated. Because of the presence of synergistic nutrients, the vitamins and minerals in whole foods are much more useful to the body than isolated synthetic vitamins and minerals. However, since our "stomachs aren't big enough" to hold all the bulk that it would take to satisfy our nutrient requirements, what are we to do? We have three choices: fresh juices, vitamin and mineral supplements and/or super (green) foods. Juicing is optional, while supplemental nutrients from super foods and/or vitamin/mineral capsules/tablets are a must.

REPAIRING THE INTESTINAL MUCOSA

By now it is clear that many chronic health problems are caused by the entry of toxins into the body, many of them through the lining of the digestive tract. As noted, this lining is called the digestive mucosa or mucosal lining. When the mucosa is healthy, it will prevent toxins (and parasites, yeasts, etc.) from entering the body. When it is unhealthy, these toxins are allowed to travel freely into the bloodstream, and from there they circulate throughout the body. This condition is called "leaky gut," and may lead to many chronic disorders. Therefore, one of the most important things we can do to achieve vibrant health is to repair the mucosa and keep it in a healthy condition. There are some simple steps that can be taken to help heal and maintain this all-important digestive lining.

The lining of the digestive tract becomes porous as the result of many different factors. Foods to which we are allergic or sensitive can be either the result or the cause of leaky gut.

Some of the other factors that adversely affect the gut lining are stress, drugs, poor diet, unhealthy lifestyle and the aging process. When the gut lining has eroded, an overabundance of free radical production causes:

- Inflammation
- Irritation
- More leaky gut

This vicious cycle must be broken, starting with the following steps:

- Manage stress more effectively.
- Change eating habits (chew food thoroughly).

- Take enzymes with meals (HCl and plant-based).
- Make diet modifications.
- Eliminate toxins (general detox).
- Eliminate candida and/or parasites.
- Take nutrient supplements.

While this may sound like a lot of work, it is a process, not a destination, and patience and trust in the process are required. We do not have to do all of this at once! Between each cleansing and detox program, there is time to work on healing the gut.

If you have any of the problems listed in figure 4, try a program of supplementation that can begin to heal the intestinal lining. Those with neuro-degenerative disorders, including senile dementia, Parkinson's disease, multiple sclerosis and Alzheimer's disease, may also benefit from such a program.

Nutrients that are needed for the healing of leaky gut include the following:

Conditions That Indicate The Need for Healing a Leaky Gut

ADD	Eczema
Joint and collagen problems	Symptoms resembling autism
Food allergies	Compromised liver function
Chronic and rheumatoid arthritis	Inflammatory bowel disease
Malnutrition	Irritable bowel syndrome
Chronic fatigue	Symptoms like schizophrenia
Multiple chemical sensitivities	Skin disorders (ranging from uticaria to acne and dermatitis)[6]
Psoriasis	
Diabetes	
Fibromyalgia	

Figure 4

L-glutamine (or glutamine) – Human studies show that L-glutamine is an essential nutrient for the cells of the small intestine. It is their primary metabolic fuel. Glutamine deficiency has been shown to result in significant functional changes in the gastrointestinal tract. Dietary deficiency of glutamine is associated with atrophy and degeneration of the small intestine. Glutamine supplementation has been shown to prevent and repair damage to the intestinal mucosa due to starvation, injury, infection, immunosuppression, chemotherapy, radiation and chronic alcoholism. Studies show that L-glutamine helps to promote healing of injured gut mucosa. In a double blind human study, 24 of 57 ulcer patients were given 1.6 grams of glutamine per day. After four weeks, 22 of the 24 patients (92%) receiving glutamine showed complete healing based on symptoms and radiographic analysis.[1] Glutamine is a very important nutrient for the healing of leaky gut and should be included in a healing protocol. Dosages range from one gram to 30 grams per day, but the average therapeutic dose is approximately five grams per day. It is best taken in powdered form; taking an equivalent dose in capsule form would not be feasible, as it would require ingestion of too many capsules. L-glutamine has no taste and is easy to take.

N-aceytl-glucosamine (NAG) – Human studies show that NAG is a highly active growth promoter for *Bifobacterium bifidum*.[2] Separate but related "in vitro" animal studies demonstrate that the presence of NAG can effectively block the adherence of *Candida albicans* to the gastrointestinal mucosa.[3] NAG is usually included in well-formulated powdered glutamine supplements.

Gamma oryzanol – is derived from red rice bran. Gamma oryzanol has anti-inflammatory properties that make it useful in cases of gastritis, ulcers and IBS (irritable bowel syndrome). It normalizes gastric secretions and forms a protective barrier on the mucous lining of the intestines. Clinical studies show that orally administered gamma oryzanol is effective in the treatment of a broad range of gastrointestinal disorders.[4] It has potent antioxidant activity and is a supplement of choice for leaky gut. Double blind studies in Japan showed the effectiveness of gamma oryzanol in treating inflammatory bowel disease (IBD).[5] This ingredient should be included in your glutamine powder supplement.

Cranesbill – is an herb with anti-inflammatory properties. This herb is beneficial in an intestinal rebuilding formula as an addition to L-glutamine.

The previously listed ingredients, in combination with marigold (to soothe the digestive tract) and marshmallow (to help rid the bowel of mucus), can be found in preformulated powdered form. In addition to this formula, other substances to take include:

Gamma Linolenic Acid (GLA) – is from borage seed oil and can be effective in the prevention and treatment of gastrointestinal mucosal inflammation. GLA is an essential fatty acid (EFA) that has anti-inflammatory properties. Your daily essential oil formula should contain this EFA.

DGL (deglycyrrhizinated licorice) – usually comes in the form of a chewable tablet that can be taken before meals. It is very soothing to the upper digestive tract and may help promote healing of leaky gut.

A good supplement would include DGL, as well as aloe (for its soothing and healing effect) and glutamine (to help repair the gut lining). All of these ingredients are important keys for healing leaky gut. ✳

Notes

[1] Amber Ackerman, N.D., *Nutritional Management of Intestinal Permeability Defects.*

[2] Ibid.

[3] Ibid.

[4] Ibid.

[5] Ibid.

[6] Trent W. Nichols, M.D., and Nancy Faags, MSW, MPH *Optimal Nutrition*, Quill, 2000, p. 63.

H.O.P.E.
PROBIOTICS

SUPPLEMENT RECOMMENDATIONS

For health maintenance, we recommend taking a probiotic supplement with 5-15 billion cultures of probiotics of the *lactobaccilus* and *bifidobacterium* families. For those who are taking (or have recently taken) antibiotics and those with health challenges, we recommend a probiotic supplement with 50 billion cultures per capsule. Look for one that has a delivery system to allow the cultures to survive stomach acid. Eating yogurt with live cultures can also help supplement beneficial bacteria.

The basic functions of the digestive system have long been understood. However, the body of scientific information on the intestinal environment and its link to disease and aging continues to grow. It is now known that a healthy, balanced digestive environment is a cornerstone of vibrant health. Conversely, an imbalanced digestive sysem can lead to chronic disease and reduced life expectancy.

As we expand our knowledge of what constitutes a healthy digestive environment, it becomes clear that many of the health problems commonly associated with aging are closely related to an imbalance in the intestinal chemistry and microbial flora. The next step, as practitioners, is to learn how we can better understand the intestinal environment, and how to help our patients achieve longevity and better health through digestive care and a balanced intestinal environment.

Brenda Watson, N.D., C.T., and Leonard Smith, M.D., *The Advanced Guide to Longevity Medicine*

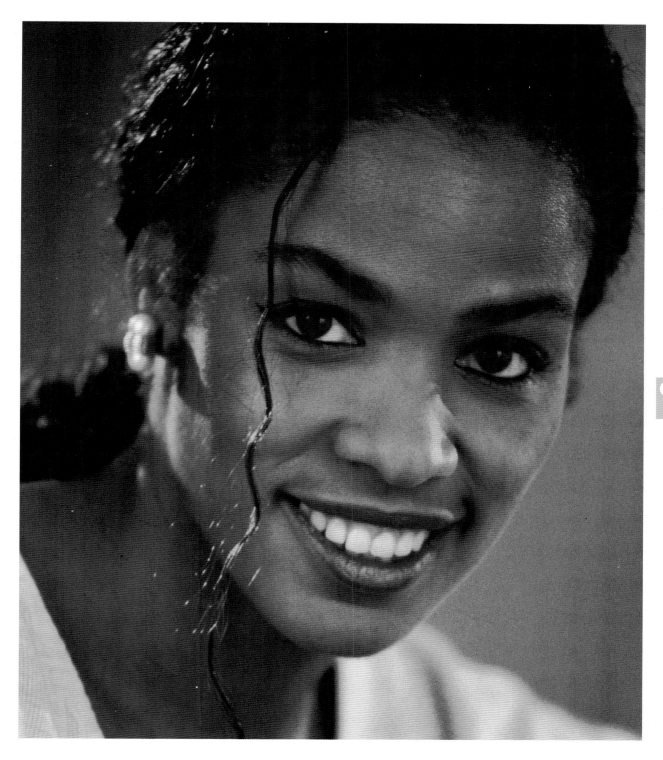

6

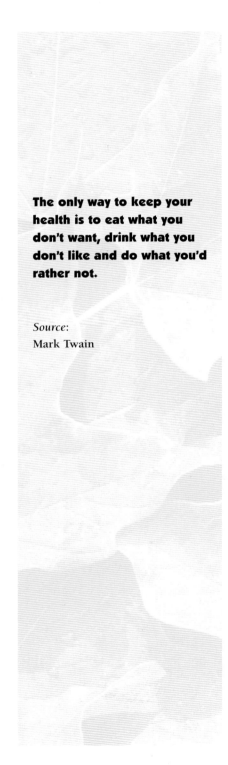

The only way to keep your health is to eat what you don't want, drink what you don't like and do what you'd rather not.

Source:
Mark Twain

CHAPTER 7

H.O.P.E.

enzymes TAKEN WITH MEALS

This chapter presents guidelines to enhance the digestive process, the first step in the prevention of disease as aging occurs. Whether we experience minor symptoms like fatigue or heartburn or already have such conditions as fibromyalgia or irritable bowel syndrome, the process of healing and restoring the body to health involves taking certain steps. Maintaining good health requires wise choices. Health is not just the absence of disease or pain. Holistic health is defined in terms of the whole person, not in terms of diseased body parts. It encompasses the psychological, mental, emotional, social, spiritual and environmental aspects of the individual. Health is a continuum, with optimal health at one end, and toxic overload, which may manifest as cancer, autoimmune disease or some other form of disease or disability, at the opposite end. Optimal health is a dynamic process that is always moving in one direction or the other on this continuum (see figure 1).

A proactive approach is required to achieve optimal health regardless of where a person's health is located on the continuum. People who feel good are less likely to believe they need to take preventive measures such as cleansing (detoxification) programs or adding digestive enzymes to their diet. These are a must in today's world because no one is totally protected. People who are experiencing toxic overload (bottom of the continuum) are usually in pain. They often reach for a more holistic approach when modern medicine no longer seems to work. These people must begin to take responsibility and action if health is to be regained to any degree!

The process of restoring wellness to the body begins by creating a lifelong maintenance/prevention program. If people hold steadfast to this goal once health has been restored, then they will increase the chances of being free of pain and the need for medication.

As "The Healing Process" (figure 2) indicates, managing stress and enhancing digestion are the second steps toward vibrant health.

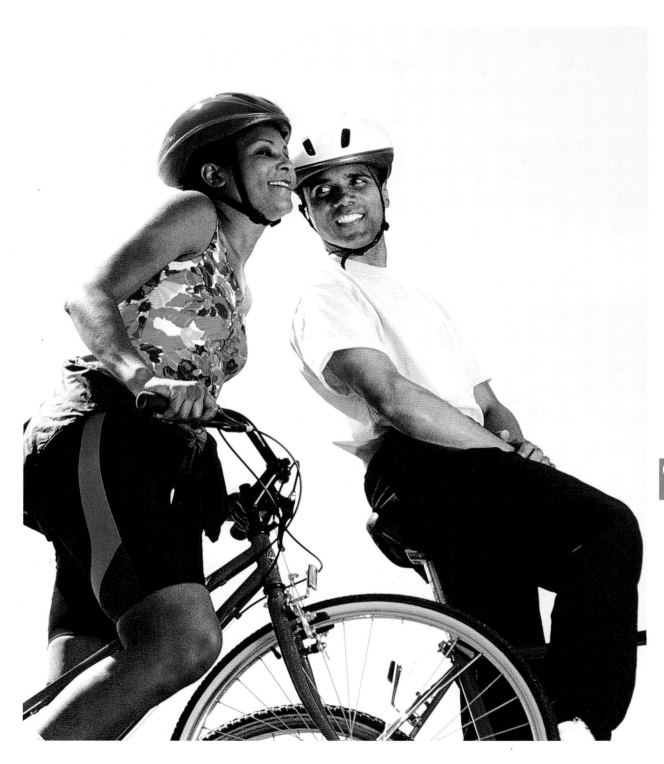

7

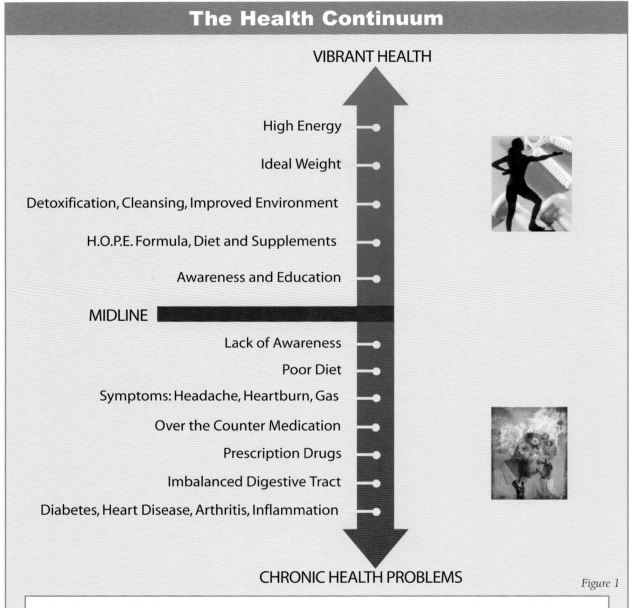

The Health Continuum

VIBRANT HEALTH

High Energy

Ideal Weight

Detoxification, Cleansing, Improved Environment

H.O.P.E. Formula, Diet and Supplements

Awareness and Education

MIDLINE

Lack of Awareness

Poor Diet

Symptoms: Headache, Heartburn, Gas

Over the Counter Medication

Prescription Drugs

Imbalanced Digestive Tract

Diabetes, Heart Disease, Arthritis, Inflammation

CHRONIC HEALTH PROBLEMS

Figure 1

Health is more than lack of symptoms. To maintain or regain it requires awareness, commitment, discipline and adherence to a proactive program emphasizing detoxification and rebuilding through diet and supplementation. The net result will be high levels of energy and a sense of well-being.

The road to chronic disease and disability, on the other hand, begins with lack of awareness, poor diet and symptom suppression through use of pharmaceutical drugs. Here the stage is set for the development of digestive dysfunction, which increases the body's toxic load and depletes its energy. The net result is development of more and more symptoms, leading ultimately to degenerative disease.

Manage Stress

The balance of mental, emotional and spiritual health in any individual is extremely important. Stress comes in many forms, and it is important to identify the source(s). Stress often stems from problems with relationships, work and/or finances.

How do you find relief from stressful situations that occur in life? It depends on your everyday choices. For example, after a stressful day at work, do you take a walk, or stop at a bar for a few drinks?

The digestive system, as noted, is very sensitive to stress levels. The capability of the organs to produce enzymes can be adversely affected by stress. As stress continues, there is a notable increase in intestinal permeability, which can allow for the absorption of undigested food. Chapter 2 dealt with food sensitivities, and how undigested food particles enter the bloodstream through the bowel wall (leading to an allergic response). The body reacts with antibody production against

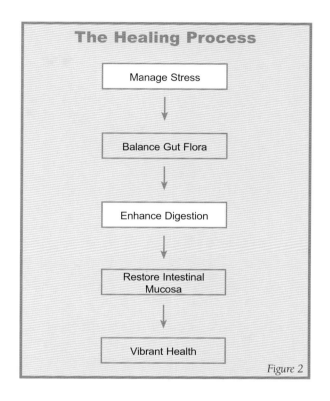

Figure 2

the undigested food because it is identified as "foreign." During *any* stress response, we go into sympathetic dominance, and digestion suffers, because blood and energy are diverted away from the digestive organs toward the skeletal muscles and brain—preparing the body for fight or flight. Eating should never occur in such a state. If it does, the food will not be digested, and an allergic reaction or sensitivity to it may well develop.

Regardless of degree of hunger, it is best to forgo eating until the stress response subsides or is consciously eliminated. Such conscious control can be learned by practicing techniques for relaxation of the body and mind. These techniques may involve the practice of meditation and/or relaxation exercises, physical exercises and deep breathing. Spending "quiet time" alone, perhaps in a serene outdoor environment, may help reduce stress, as may listening to soothing music or recordings

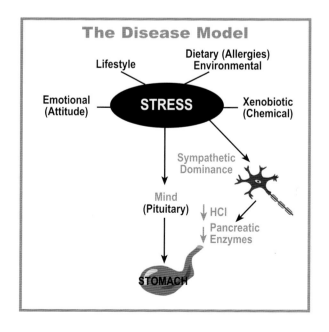

7

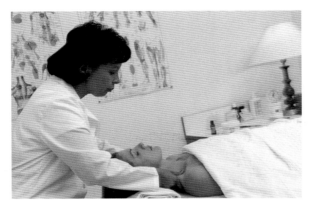

of nature sounds. Warm baths can be relaxing, as can massages. The practice of "giving thanks" and maintaining a moment of silence before eating is one that is certainly conducive to relaxation and thus to good digestion as well.

It has been discovered fairly recently that the bowel wall has a "mind of its own," so to speak, in that it actually contains the same receptors as the brain and undergoes similar neurological processes, especially with regard to serotonin receptors. Essentially then, the bowel quite literally makes "decisions" with regard to absorption and motility. These decisions, like decisions made by the brain, can be hugely influenced by our emotional state.

There are additional steps to take to create a more harmonious lifestyle and relieve stress when the need arises. Important considerations in the management of stress are lifestyle factors such as time management and exercise.

Helpful time management practices include:

• Setting priorities – be realistic in what can be accomplished.
• Creating a definite eating plan for the week.
• Organizing the day.

Exercise is of utmost importance in managing stress. As we exercise, we become stronger. The body functions more efficiently and develops greater endurance. Exercise also helps regulate blood sugar levels, so that energy is more sustained during the day. It helps the brain release **endorphins** (morphine-like substances) that can lead to a euphoric or happy feeling. Exercise has been also shown to increase the blood levels of phenylethylamine, the chemical that is released when humans are in love! Exercise should be enjoyable, not a forced activity. Walking, yoga and biking, even though dissimilar activities, can all create the same sense of well being in a person and definitely help in creating better digestion, absorption and assimilation of nutrients from food.

ENHANCE DIGESTION

Enhanced digestion is the next step in the healing process. This requires:

• Following dietary guidelines
• Chewing foods thoroughly
• Eating consciously
• Eating a variety of foods
• Following food-combining rules if digestion is compromised
• Supplementation with plant enzymes and HCl (hydrochloric acid) for better digestion

Following dietary guidelines certainly challenges most people in today's fast-paced environment, but it is decidedly the most critical component of healing and preventive health care.

There are many misunderstandings about food and nutrition. Even experts in the field of health can become confused: One day eggs are good; the next day they are reported to be bad. Fiber is deemed good for lowering cholesterol and helping to prevent colon cancer, and then its benefits are questioned. Depending upon who's doing and reporting the research, there will always be conflicting findings. The real challenge is finding the right balance. This comes with moderation and common sense. Excessive amounts of sugar and refined foods are very bad, not only for the digestive system, but also for the immune system.

Thorough Chewing

Digestion begins in the mouth. If food is not chewed thoroughly, the amylase enzymes from the saliva aren't in contact with it long enough to begin the digestive process. When large bits of insufficiently chewed food move to the stomach, we may experience gas or indigestion. Eating too rapidly can cause bloating because excessive air is ingested. Many people chew their food only a couple of times before washing it down with water or some other beverage. This results in dilution of digestive juices and further digestive stress. Digestion can be improved by simply taking more time to thoroughly chew food, so that the first phase of carbohydrate digestion functions properly.

Eating on the run or making meal time social time, can divert attention from the eating (and chewing) process. If food is typically chewed less than 10 times before swallowing, then a concerted effort should be made to extend chewing time. Try chewing food as much as 30 times so that it is liquefied. The more thoroughly it is chewed, the better the digestive process will function.

Conscious eating is another important factor to ensure proper digestion of food. To support good digestion, the "conscious" eater will want to:

• Prepare an enjoyable atmosphere for eating (not in the car).
• Eat in a relaxed atmosphere.
• Eat at a moderate pace. Slow down!

Cold liquids or excessive liquid intake should be avoided during meals. Cold beverages slow the digestive process. Too much liquid during meals dilutes enzymes, interrupting the digestive

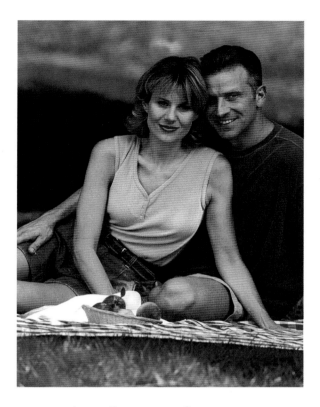

process. A small amount of room temperature liquid with meals (tea/water) is okay, as is taking supplements with water after meals.

Variety is the spice of life, and the body knows this instinctively. Eating the same foods again and again, day after day (especially processed foods), can increase food sensitivities. A rotation of foods, which reduces repetitive eating habits, is best.

Enzyme Supplementation

Historically, the best sources of enzymes have been from the consumption of fresh fruits and vegetables. Eating these foods on a daily basis is the foundation of good health. Even the food pyramid requires three to five servings of vegetables and two to three servings of fruit daily. Unfortunately, too many people disregard these daily guidelines.

7

Enzymes are essential for all chemical processes in the body, including digestion. The enzymatic level of fresh foods, such as fruits and vegetables, is reduced by long-term storage and pesticides and toxins in the water and soil. As we age, the number of enzymes and their activity levels decrease. This is why supplementation with enzymes is helpful.

Cooking food destroys enzymes, which are needed for virtually every chemical reaction in the body. For this reason, a diet that is at least 50% raw is recommended. However, we still have the problem of enzyme destruction with the 50% of the food that's cooked. The obvious solution is to use enzyme supplements. People with digestive problems will want to take digestive enzymes with every meal. Others may do so as well—or take them just with cooked meals.

A good enzyme supplement will not just substitute for the body in the digestive process: Supplementing with digestive enzymes will decrease the need for all of the pancreatic enzyme secretions to be active in the digestive tract. This will allow some of the pancreatic enzymes to be absorbed into the blood where they can work on that portion of food that enters the blood and lymphatic system undigested, helping to break it down. Pancreatic enzymes also enhance the immune system.

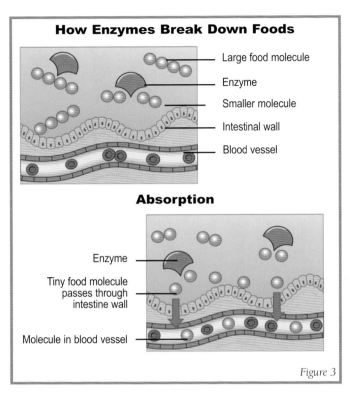

How Enzymes Break Down Foods

- Large food molecule
- Enzyme
- Smaller molecule
- Intestinal wall
- Blood vessel

Absorption

- Enzyme
- Tiny food molecule passes through intestine wall
- Molecule in blood vessel

Figure 3

A good digestive enzyme formula will contain a variety of enzymes to address every type of food group ingested: fats, starches, dairy, plant, vegetable material (cellulose) and sugar. The ideal digestive enzyme supplement would be plant-based. Such enzymes are already activated as they enter the system and therefore start to work in the stomach, continuing to function throughout the body with a broad pH range, from 2 to 14. When digestion is incomplete, plant enzymes act like "Pac Man,™" breaking down and cleaning up undigested food in the digestive tract. This undigested food gives rise to toxin production in the intestinal tract, which would eventually lead to toxic overload.

Plant enzymes are the best choice for indigestion or as a preventive measure to ensure complete digestion. Anyone older than 40 should have plant enzymes in their daily regimen. It is also a good choice for people younger than 40, and for

Q. Will plant enzymes stop my digestive organs from producing their own enzymes?

A. No. Plant enzymes simply support your digestive process.

> Fewer than 10 percent of Americans eat 2 servings of fruit or 3 servings of vegetables daily. Fifty percent eat no vegetables at all, 70 percent eat no vegetables or fruits rich in vitamin C, and 80 percent eat no vegetables or fruits rich in carotenoids per day.

vegetarians. Plant enzymes can be taken at higher doses by people who have microbial infections (especially parasites) in the intestinal tract. These enzymes may be used by people with lower gastric (stomach) distress: bloating, flatulence and cramping. Take one to three capsules with, or directly following, each meal.

People older than 40 who are deficient in HCl may address that deficiency by taking a HCl supplement. Those with candida can also benefit from a HCl supplement, for they often have low levels of stomach acid. Those experiencing upper gastric distress—heartburn, reflux or belching—could benefit from taking products with HCl as well. HCl will prevent bacterial invasion by killing bacteria entering the mouth and stomach. A HCl-containing digestive formula is recommended while traveling to help prevent this invasion of bacteria.

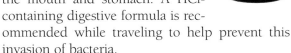
Plant Enzymes

If you are not sure you have low stomach acid, refer to the symptoms in Chapter 2. A stool test can also be done to detect the presence of undigested meat fibers. (See Resource Directory lab listing). One way to determine if you are producing sufficient HCl is to take 600-800mgs. of HCl on an empty stomach a few minutes before a meal. If, after a few minutes, you feel a warm sensation in your stomach, you are producing

sufficient stomach acid. If no warming occurs, take another capsule, and continue to take one every 15 minutes until warming occurs. Once stomach is warm, determine how many capsules you have taken, and subtract one. This is the correct dosage for you to take with meals. The amount of food eaten at a meal can also be a factor in how much HCl is needed. Once diet and health improve, less HCl is needed, and plant enzymes become the primary support for digestion.

> Look for quality plant enzyme products that have high levels of protease and contain lipase, amylase, lactase, cellulase and invertase (for sugar). A good formula will also include ingredients like glutamine and gamma oryzanol to help support the lining of the digestive tract. A blend of herbs like ginger, marshmallow, bromelain and papaya should also be included in the formula. This type of enzyme mix is formulated for people who want to receive more nutritional value from the foods they eat.

A good HCl supplement might also contain pepsin, quercitin, bromelain, butryric acid, N-acetyl-glucosamine, L-glutamine, gamma oryzanol and other soothing ingredients.

Some people with gastritis or heartburn can have *too much* stomach acid as a result of diet or stress. DGL (deglycyrrhizinated licorice) is a good choice for these people. Chewable DGL is taken before meals to soothe the stomach. It helps the cells of the stomach by improving the blood supply (and bringing nutrients to it). A good formula contains not only the DGL but also aloe and L-glutamine. Aloe is soothing to the mucosal lining, and

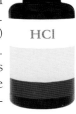
HCl

7

L-glutamine helps restore this lining.

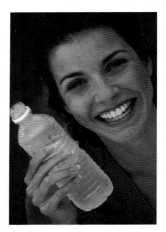

Those experiencing upper abdominal distress (heartburn, reflux or belching) may have an imbalance in their stomach. These symptoms can occur with too much acid, normal acid or even low acid in the stomach. Although this statement may appear contradictory, these different acid levels can cause the same symptoms. Dehydration can cause *any* amount of acid to irritate the stomach. When people do not drink enough water, the mucous lining that is produced to protect the stomach from acid can be damaged and hampered in its ability to regenerate. A good rule of thumb is to drink a glass of room temperature water 30 minutes before a meal to protect and nourish the mucous lining so it can regenerate at regular intervals.

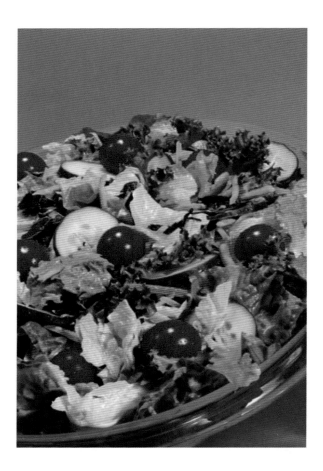

Acid irritation, combined with poor gastric digestion, can cause distention, as well as reflux of food into the esophagus, which does not have the protective lining to deal with the acid. When such acid irritation occurs, HCl may be worth a trial because it can kill bacteria and help gastric protein digestion. This regimen, with the addition of digestive enzymes, aloe, DGL and glutamine, often completely relieves upper abdominal symptoms when combined with the right eating habits. It may be helpful, for a short period of time, to use acid blockers, but long-term use of antacids create significant problems with digestion and microbial overgrowth, especially *H. pylori*, the bacterium that causes gastric and duodenal ulcers.

H.O.P.E.

ENZYMES

SUPPLEMENT RECOMMENDATIONS

For those with low levels of stomach acid, we recommend a plant-based digestive enzyme formula that contains HCl. For general digestive support, as well as for those who have digestive difficulty and suffer from gas and bloating, we recommend a high potency plant-based blend that contains enzymes to assist in the breakdown of protein, carbohydrates, fats, sugars and fiber.

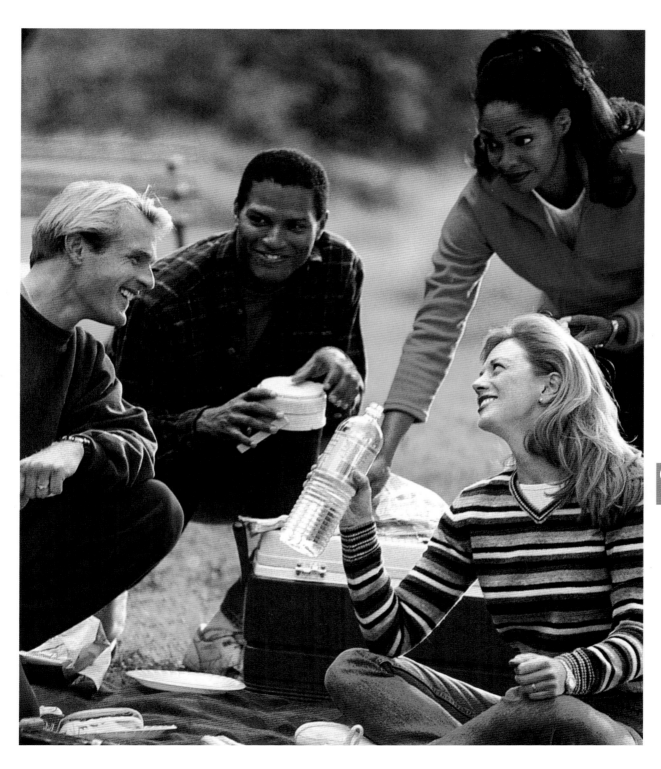

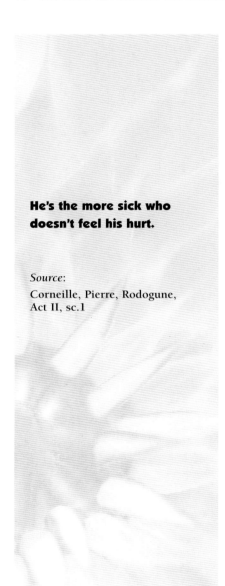

CHAPTER 8

DIETARY GUIDELINES FOR
health MAINTENANCE

The first step toward improved health is to eat fresh, clean, whole foods —foods in their natural state that have not been commercially processed. Sounds simple enough, but, sadly, eating a "good diet," or even knowing just what constitutes one, is not simple at all in today's "fast food" world.

There are many myths about healthy food selection and preparation. It is the goal of this chapter to dispel some of those myths and describe exactly what constitutes a "good diet." Understand that what's being described here is a good *basic* diet, one which will help *prevent*, not treat, disease—though adhering to these dietary principles may well result in the disappearance of some unpleasant symptoms. The "diet" described here is not really so much a diet as it is a lifestyle, a way of eating.

You'll recall from Chaper 2 that many causes of impaired digestion have to do with our eating habits—what, how and/or when we eat. In this chaper, we'll look at how to develop healthy eating habits that will aid the digestion process rather than inhibit it.

The components of a healthy diet are organized under these subtopics:

• Time Management and Meal Planning
• Whole Foods vs. Processed Foods
• Balancing Proteins, Starches and Fats
• pH Balancing
• Raw Foods vs. Cooked Foods
• The Importance of Oils, Nuts and Seeds
• The Role of Fiber, Beans, Grains
• Portion Control
• Vegetarian vs. Non-Vegetarian Diets
• Nutrient Supplementation

Time Management and Meal Planning

Meal planning and time management are key components in creating

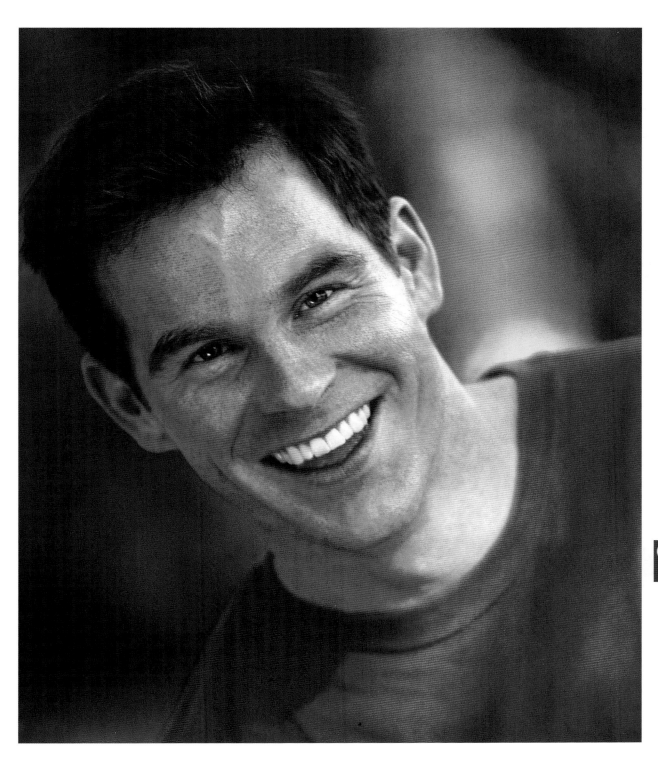

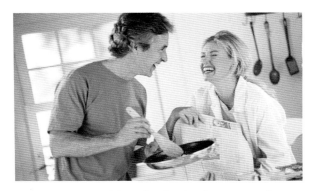

a healthy eating plan, for food selection is of paramount importance in achieving vibrant health. The first step is reviewing your lifestyle and determining how healthy foods can be integrated into it. Plan your meals for one week before visiting the market. When possible, plan lunches for you and your children ahead of time. Typical school lunches are not very nourishing, and neither are the fast foods so popular at lunch. Ideally, meal planning for the coming week would be done on the weekend or on your day off. Selections would best be written down for better organizing and planning. Make grocery shopping a part of your weekly routine, and make a habit of washing fruits and vegetables thoroughly before storing them. This saves time during the week when time is of the essence. If a weekly plan includes eating at restaurants, then select only those that offer healthy options.

Local markets and health food stores offer the best choices of quality foods to be prepared at home. Look for stores that stock organic fruits, vegetables and meats. You'll want to discard any unhealthy foods—sugar, refined starches, soda pop, etc.—that may have been purchased before starting your healthy diet.

Looking at what you will need in terms of appliances will save you time in the kitchen. One of the most important time-saving appliances is the crock-pot. With it, foods are cooked slowly throughout the day and are ready to serve when you get home from work.

Whole Foods vs. Processed

Any food that is not "whole" is fragmented, and that fragmentation occurs as the result of food processing procedures designed to extend shelf life and make the food look fresh and attractive. These processes include enriching, homogenizing, flavoring, preserving, milling, pasteurizing, coloring, irradiating, emulsifying, thickening, stabilizing, hydrogenating, etc. While these processes may enhance the appearance of the foods and make them last longer, they do so at the expense of nutrients. Many food processing procedures involve the application of heat, which destroys enzymes, as well as many vitamins and minerals.

 **VS.**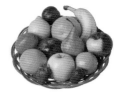

Focusing on fresh fruits and vegetables, preferably organic ones, is recommended when making the transition from processed to whole foods. Agricultural use of pesticides and herbicides has escalated wildly during a relatively brief span of time. Amazingly, as many as 60 cancer-causing pesticides can be legally used to grow most common foods.[1] In 1993, a study conducted by the Environmental Working Group concluded that, by age five, children have consumed more pesticides than considered safe for a lifetime. These pesticides are fat-soluble, so they cannot be washed off the produce (and are retained in the body). Ingesting them puts a tremendous strain on the detoxification systems of the liver. In today's world, it's imperative to "go organic" to retain or regain health. Washing organic produce in either hydrogen peroxide or a special "veggie wash" solution is very important, for these foods are apt to carry parasites. Organic dairy and meat products are wise choices as well, since today's "factory farm" animals are often diseased and loaded with antibiotics and growth hormones.

If fresh organic produce is unavailable, select frozen over canned. It has more nutritional value. Be sure to read labels, and avoid those foods that list chemical preservatives. Also, avoid added sugar and artificial sweeteners, especially aspartame. It is a "neurotoxic substance that has been associated with numerous health problems including dizziness, visual impairment, severe muscle aches, numbing of extremities, high blood pressure, retinal hemorrhaging, seizures and depression."[2] Other foods to avoid are those containing "partially hydrogenated vegetable oil." This man-made oil is found in commercial peanut butter, margarine and most baked goods. Most supermarket oils are refined (unless kept in a special "health food" section) and not so labeled. Make sure the oil you use is labeled "unrefined" or "expeller pressed."

Most packaged grains found in grocery stores are refined. White rice is an example. Choose brown rice over white. Try some of the less familiar but highly nourishing whole grains like millet, buckwheat, teff, quinoa, amaranth, spelt, bulgur wheat and barley. These are all available, often in bulk form, through natural food stores. You'll want to "go organic" with these foods, as well as others, whenever possible.

Balancing Proteins, Carbohydrates and Fats

Macronutrients consist of proteins, fats and carbohydrates (simple ones like fruit and "starchy" ones like grains). Our general health, it seems, is influenced by the percentage of caloric intake from each of these groups. There is compelling evidence that the high-carbohydrate/low-fat diet, once touted as the ideal, has some undesirable effects on health: weight gain, hypoglycemia (low blood sugar) and heart disease. Researchers have found that such

an eating plan is deficient in essential fatty acids, and the low protein-to-carbohydrate ratio results in excessive insulin release (when refined carbohydrates are eaten) and inhibition of the hormone **glucagon** (when protein is eaten). The net effect of the high-carb/low-fat diet is fat storage (weight gain), lowering of blood sugar levels and hormonal imbalances (from essential fatty acid deficiencies).

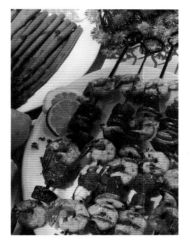

Dr. Barry Sears, a pioneer researcher in this field, has proposed a solution to this potential problem: the 40/30/30 eating plan (40% of calories from carbohydrates, 30% from protein and 30% from fat). This balanced eating plan avoids the problems associated with the high-carbohydrate/low-fat diet. However, calculating the percentage of calories from each macronutrient for each meal can be time-consuming and somewhat problematic. A simpler method is to watch (and, if necessary, limit) refined carbohydrate intake. Also, make sure that the protein food in a meal is about the size of the palm of your hand, and add olive oil to salads.

pH Balancing

What's important to know about pH (acidity/alkalinity) is that most grains, all meats and sugary foods are acid-forming in the body, while most fruits (even citrus) and vegetables are alkaline-forming (though they may be acid in their raw, undigested form). The consensus among experts in the natural health field seems to be that the ideal diet would consist of 80% alkaline-forming foods, 20% acid-forming foods. That means more fruits and vegetables should be eaten than meats and grains. The SAD (Standard American Diet) is backwards, with emphasis on starchy carbohydrates and meat. This imbalance can be corrected by adding fruits and vegetables to the diet while limiting starchy carbohydrates.

A green salad at least once per day and at least one cooked green vegetable daily, gradually adding more greens, will achieve an ideal diet. In addition to increasing the number of salads and vegetables eaten, you may wish to add green drinks and/or capsules to your daily routine. See Resource Directory for specific products.

Raw Foods vs. Cooked Foods

Chapter 2 emphasized that enzymes are destroyed by 116 degrees or more of heat. Since meats are generally prepared at a temperature of at least 350 degrees and grains at 325 degrees and more, wholesale enzyme destruction occurs when these foods are cooked. Any processed foods, even uncooked, are devoid of enzymes due to the heat applied in the refining process. Freezing and refrigeration also have some effect on enzymes but result in only about a 30% loss.

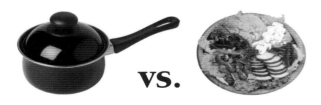

Enzymes are actually proteins. They consist of amino acids and are the body's building blocks. When enzymes in food are destroyed or reduced, the digestive organs have to work harder to break down and process that food. Metabolic enzymes are then forced to perform this function instead of their intended job of healing. A deficiency of enzymes in the body is synonymous with a deficiency of life force.

Nothing shows the value of raw foods more than the work done by the late Francis Pottenger, M.D. In 1946, he experimented with 900 cats. Half were fed raw milk and raw meat; the other half ate cooked meat and pasteurized (cooked) milk. During a 10-year period, he found that the cats on the raw diet thrived, while those on the cooked food diet showed all the degenerative diseases common in man. By the third generation, all the cats on the processed diet were sterile or congenitally malformed.

Not only do we have more energy (life force) from raw foods in our diet, but our bodies are more thoroughly hydrated due to their high water content. A diet of exclusively cooked foods forces the body to use its own fluids to moisten the ingested food, and it therefore has a dehydrating effect. Dehydration is an important, though often overlooked, cause of many disorders, including constipation. Those with raw foods in their diet will require less extra water intake than those eating predominantly cooked foods.

Any food prepared at temperatures less than 116 degrees may be considered "raw." Although conventional cooking requires much higher temperatures, tasty foods can be prepared at extremely low temperatures or without heat, using kitchen appliances such as juicers, dehydrators, food processors and blenders. There are many fine "cook" books available at natural foods stores on how to prepare tasty raw foods.

Add raw foods gradually to your diet, especially if your current diet is composed largely of cooked food and/or you suffer from digestive disorders. Some people with inflammatory conditions can't

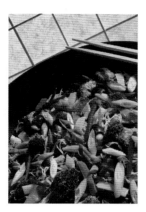

process raw foods, or in some extreme cases, even cooked vegetables. Each person is different and must do what is best for his or her unique body chemistry. The simplest way to add raw foods is to alter cooking methods. As healing of the digestive tract occurs and as tolerance permits, less and less cooked foods are required. For example, the steaming time on vegetables may be gradually reduced so that they're eventually firm instead of soft, or they may be stir-fried to a similar consistency. Vegetables should never be boiled. Experiment to see what you can tolerate. If vegetables are a problem, you may supplement with green drinks or capsules. (See Resource Directory.)

The Importance of Oils, Nuts and Seeds

Oils are actually fats, one of the three macronutrients noted earlier. While people concerned with weight loss are conditioned to view fat as a foe, the truth is that good health and normal weight cannot be maintained without an adequate amount of good quality fat in the diet.

There are three types of fats: **saturated, monounsaturated** and **polyunsaturated**. Saturation refers to the way that hydrogen is carried in the fatty acid molecule and to the number of hydrogen bonds in the chemical structure of the fatty acid. Saturated fats include all meat fats, dairy products, palm and coconut oil and the man-made hydrogenated oils. Monounsaturated fatty acids are found in olive oil, canola oil and peanut oil. The polyunsaturates are further divided into the EFAs omega-3 and omega-6. The best known sources of the omega-6s are borage, evening primrose oil and black currant seed oil. Fish oils and flax oil

feature a high content of omega-3 fatty acids.

To maintain health, the body needs a balance of all these types of oil. Problems arise when too much of any given type of fat is consumed. The Western diet has, during the last hundred years, favored fats from meat and dairy products and vegetable seed oils. This has disrupted the balance between omega-3 and omega-6 fatty acids. This balance can be restored by eating more omega-3-rich fats from fish, vegetables, flax oil and walnuts.

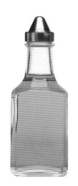

Many have heard of the "dangers" of saturated fat from meat. There is nothing dangerous about saturated fat. This form of fat is needed, but in excess it becomes a problem. The same is true of the other natural fats. We've also heard from the media about the detrimental effects of coconut and palm oils. There seems to be no basis for these rumors; in fact, all of the tropical oils contain large amounts of **lauric acid**, which has strong anti-fungal and anti-microbial properties.[3] Furthermore, these oils have a very high "flash point," meaning they can withstand high temperatures without becoming rancid. They are therefore excellent cooking oils. Sesame oil and butter may likewise be used for cooking. While flax is an excellent source of omega-3, it is very heat-sensitive and so should not come into contact with heat. This is also true of safflower oil, unless it is the "high oleic" variety. The only fats to

8

Fats serve many vital functions in the body. They:

- **Facilitate oxygen transport**
- **Lubricate and insulate muscles and organs**
- **Aid in the absorption of fat-soluble vitamins**
- **Nourish the skin, mucous membranes and nerves**
- **Help maintain body temperature**

avoid totally are the hydrogenated ones and canola oil. Hydrogenated oil is a man-made oil that the body cannot metabolize.

Canola oil has become very popular today, though there has been much controversy surrounding it. Canola oil comes from the rapeseed plant, which has a very high content of **erucic acid**. Rat studies have found erucic acid to cause fatty degeneration of the heart and other organs. Based on these studies, "canola" oil was bred as a special strain of **rapeseed** that contains a very low amount of erucic acid. Ironically however, it was later found that rats do not metabolize fats and oils well, so that *any* type of oil would be damaging to them.[4] Does this mean then that canola oil may be consumed safely by humans? Maybe not. It seems that this oil is high in sulfur and becomes rancid easily, so that baked goods made with it produce mold quickly. Processed canola oil also contains trans fats, which can be damaging to the body.[5] Considering these findings, it may be wise to just avoid the use of canola oil.

The important things to know about oils are to use unrefined ones and *refrigerate them*. Refrigeration is actually optional for the tropical oils but a necessity with other types of oil since they spoil readily when exposed to heat and light. Air exposure will also cause these oils to spoil, so they should be tightly sealed. You will also want to refrigerate nuts and seeds, and, since they contain enzyme inhibitors, which make them difficult to digest, they should be soaked overnight in water to make them more digestible.

Portion Control

Because overeating can put stress on the digestive organs and lead to obesity and disease, many of us would do well to address the issue of portion control. Sometimes the food portions on eating guidelines are not easy to calculate without a scale or measuring device. Therefore, the following guidelines for determining size are suggested:

- **1 ounce of American cheese** slightly larger than a standard 3.5-inch computer diskette

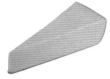

- **3 ounces of cooked lean meat** the size of the palm of a woman's hand or the size of a deck of cards

- **1/2 cup of cooked pasta** smaller than the base of a computer mouse (2 1/2-inch long, 1 1/4-inch high)

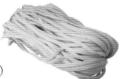

- **a 2-inch standard square brownie** about the size of a business card

- **a slice of pizza (1/12 of a large pie)** should fit inside a standard business envelope

- **2 tablespoons of salad dressing** would fill 1/6th of a standard 6-ounce paper cup from the water cooler

- **a 4-ounce bagel** about the size of a compact disc

The following list helps to decipher serving sizes often found in food guidelines like the Food Guide Pyramid. (This information, and the previous, was taken from http://www.thriveonline.aol.com/nutrition/experts/joan/joan.10-27-98.html):

Bread. . . . . one slice
Cereal . . . . 1 ounce ready-to-eat
Cooked cereal. . . . . 1/2 cup
Rice. . . . . 1/2 cup cooked

Pasta . . . . 1/2 cup cooked
Raw, leafy vegetables. . . . 1 cup
   chopped, raw
   or cooked . . . . 1/2 cup
Vegetable juice . . . . 3/4 cup
Whole fruit . . . . one medium
   chopped, cooked or
   canned fruit. . . . . 1/2 cup
100% fruit juice . . . . 3/4 cup
Milk . . . . 1 cup
Yogurt . . . . 1 cup
Natural cheese . . . . 1 1/2 ounces
Processed cheese. . . . . . 2 ounces

Vegetarian vs. Non-Vegetarian Diets

Virtually all *cleansing* diets eliminate meat. During times of cleansing, this difficult-to-digest, fiber-less food is often best replaced by more digestible, high-fiber vegetables or by a juice diet with supplemental fiber. While an unsupervised juice diet should not exceed five days, one can safely eliminate meat from the diet for an extended period of time with no ill effects, making for a prolonged cleanse. Improvement in various disorders, including arthritis, kidney disease, skin disorders and gout, have been reported as the result of following a meatless diet. However, many people who have followed strict vegetarian diets and benefited from them initially have found that, after a time, their health declined and did not improve until meat was returned to their diets.

Similarly, the late Weston Price, D.D.S., found, through his examination of the dental health and lifestyles of a variety of indigenous tribes throughout the world, that the healthiest were those who ate meat. Those primitive people who ate largely grains and legumes were much healthier than "civilized" people, but developed more dental caries than the primitives who subsisted primarily on meat and fish.

It would appear that in the short run we can thrive on a vegetarian diet; however, in the long run, we need some animal protein, or we risk losing the benefits gained from the cleansing effect of the meatless diet. How long can we thrive on a meatless diet before our health begins to decline? It would appear that the amount of time differs from person to person. There are many factors involved. One appears to be blood type. Much has been written about how people with different blood types have different food tolerances. The point is often made that people with type A blood are inherently low in HCl and therefore do well on a vegetarian diet. What may be more accurate is that people with blood type A need fewer animal products less often than other blood types, and/or that they may be able to subsist more comfortably and longer on a vegan (no animal products) diet than other blood types.

Another factor appears to be the country of origin of one's ancestors. Ancestors coming from tropical climates subsisted largely on tropical fruits, light meats and vegetables grown above the ground, while those from cold countries lived on heavier meats, stews and root vegetables. It has been demonstrated that

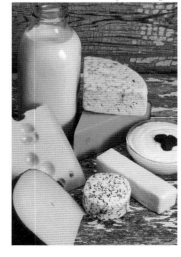

people tend to maintain better health when they stick to their indigenous diet than when they deviate from it. Yet another factor in determining the best diet for an individual is the metabolic rate (the rate at which food is converted to energy). Fast metabolizers do well with foods that take longer to digest, while the opposite is true for slow metabolizers.

Regardless of individual biochemical differences, however, it's accurate to say that *most people* 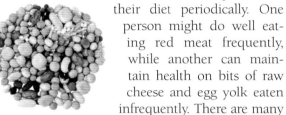 need some animal protein in their diet periodically. One person might do well eating red meat frequently, while another can maintain health on bits of raw cheese and egg yolk eaten infrequently. There are many reasons for this. Sally Fallon does an excellent job of outlining these in her section on "proteins" in *Nourishing Traditions*.[6] The points made below come directly from her book.

It is well-known that animal products are the only source of complete protein, meaning that they contain all of the essential amino acids (those not made in the body, which must be supplied through diet). All plant foods are low in three amino acids: tryptophan, cystine and threonine. Legumes and whole grains are the richest sources of non-animal protein, and, when consumed together, provide a complete protein profile (since legumes are high in lysine but low in methionine, and grains are just the reverse: high in methionine and low in lysine).

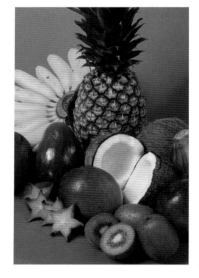

Many vegetarians eat beans as a primary protein source. While beans are composed of both proteins and carbohy-

drates, the determining factor as to which of these macronutrients will predominate is the manner in which the beans are cooked. Most cooking methods result in carbohydrate dominance. To obtain the full protein value of beans, they must first be soaked and sprouted, then cooked slowly at less than 200 degrees. A slow cooker or crock-pot works well for this purpose.

Important nutrients supplied in animal fats include the fat-soluble vitamins A and D and vitamins B6 and B12. Children vitally need these fat-soluble vitamins for their growth and development, which could be adversely affected by a vegan diet. Although the words "vegan" and "vegetarian" are being used here interchangeably, this is not technically correct. The vegan diet is a *totally* vegetarian diet, devoid of any animal products. A "vegetarian" may be vegan in his eating habits, but he *may* also include eggs (ovo-vegetarian) or milk (lacto-vegetarian) or both (ovo/lacto-vegetarian) in his diet.

While red meat is considered a "high stress" protein (takes much energy to digest) and should therefore be eaten in moderation, it is quite rich in iron and zinc, which are needed for the body's use of EFAs. It takes a strong, healthy digestive system (which most of us don't have) to tolerate a high intake of red meat. Once digestive

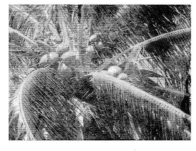

health is restored, however, most people should tolerate it in moderation. Low-stress proteins, such as poultry and fish, are ultimately the best choices.

Although animal products are essential for proper growth and development and for healthy reproduction, it is interesting that "animal studies indicate that animal protein in the amount of one sardine per person per day, combined with protein from grains and pulses [legumes], is generally sufficient to maintain reproduction and adequate growth."[7] This is encouraging for those to whom animal products have little appeal—we don't appear to need much of them in our diet to maintain health. This fact seems to relate to eating habits in the rest of the animal kingdom. Gorillas, considered to be vegetarians, eat insect eggs and larvae, as these adhere to the leaves and fruits on which the animals typically dine. So they are actually eating small amounts of animal protein.

The use of organic meats and dairy products is strongly recommended regardless of a person's choice of animal food—poultry, fish or red meat. As Fallon says of commercial meats, "According to the renowned cancer specialist, Virginia Livingston-Wheeler, most chicken, and nearly half the beef consumed in America today, is cancerous and pathogenic. Her research has convinced her that these cancers are transmissible to man."[8]

Organic meat and dairy products come from animals that have been raised without the use of antibiotics or steroids. To take things a step further, we recommend selection of milk, cheese, butter and meat that is produced from grass-fed rather than grain-fed cows. Virtually all dairy cattle live their entire lives in confinement rather than grazing in pastures as once was the norm. There is a vast difference in the health value of grass-fed vs. grain-fed beef. One major difference is in the ratio of omega-6 to omega-3 essential fatty acids. In grain-fed beef, this ratio is quite high, often approaching 20 to 1,[9] (far in excess of the 4 to 1 ratio where health problems start to surface). Grass-fed beef, on the other hand, has about the same ideal omega-6 to omega-3 ratio as fish—3 to 1.

Conjugated linoleic acid (CLA) is a naturally occurring fat that is found in abundance in hoofed animals that eat green grass, but it is greatly diminished in grain-fed animals. Grass-fed animals have three to four times more CLA than their grain-fed counterparts. This is extremely significant, for CLA has been found in animal studies to be highly protective against cancer. Human studies have also shown that CLA helps people to lose body fat while retaining muscle mass.

Unlike grain-fed animals, the grass-grazers have an abundance of fat-soluble vitamins (A & D) in their fat. Also, Dr. Weston Price discovered a fat-soluble factor that he referred to as "activator X" in butterfat from pastured cows. He found this as yet unidentified factor, which is absent in the fat of grain-fed cattle, to be a "powerful catalyst to mineral absorption."[10] The fat-soluble elements so prevalent in the butterfat of grass-fed ruminant animals also "support endocrine function, allow-

8

ing optimum physical development and lifelong good health."[11]

Grass-fed animals live longer, healthier lives than do grain-fed ones. It makes good sense therefore that humans eating products from these healthier animals would also enjoy greater health. There is a grassroots movement away from the industrialization of agriculture back to traditional farming methods. Visit www.westonaprice.org and www.eatwild.com for more information. Also see the Resource Directory in this book.

When completing a cleansing program, animal products will be the last food to be returned to the diet. How much is added and how often it is eaten is strictly a matter of personal choice.

Vegetarians (and non-vegetarians) may benefit from following the "Pro Vita Plan" developed by the late herbalist, Stuart Wheelwright, with its heavy emphasis on low-stress proteins (that take minimal energy to digest) early in the day. In the Pro Vita breakfast and lunch, five vegetables (one cooked, four raw) and five proteins (one cooked and four raw) are eaten. The raw proteins may be a mix of nuts and seeds (soaked overnight), which can be used in conjunction with a salad or mixed into a blender drink. A typical Pro Vita breakfast or lunch might look like this:

• Salad of Romaine lettuce with onions, carrots, celery, fresh basil, sprouts; dressing of soaked sesame, pumpkin and flax seeds with flax oil or olive oil/lemon/herb
• Broiled cod fish
• Steamed cauliflower

Dinner in this plan would consist of complex carbohydrates and no protein.

Nutrient Supplementation

While following a prevention program that supports longevity and vibrant health, it is a good idea to supplement with the following nutrients, as it is very difficult to obtain all the needed nutrients from food.

• High fiber from flax, gluten-free oat bran and acacia
• Essential omega-3 oils from fish
• Probiotics including acidophilus
  – After antibiotics
  – When traveling
  – During digestive upset (from food)
  – During stressful times
• Plant enzymes with meals
• Green foods (to alkalinize)
• Vitamin, mineral and antioxidant supplements after meals

These supplements are great to take every day.

Notes

[1] Carolyn DeMarco, M.D., *Breast Cancer and the Environment*, Health Counselor, vol. 8, no. 6, p. 31.

[2] Sally Fallon, *Nourishing Traditions*, New Trends Publishing, Inc., 1999, p. 51.

[3] Sally Fallon, *Nourishing Traditions*, Promotion Publishing, 1995, p. 17.

[4] Udo Erasmus, *Fats that Heal, Fats that Kill*, Alive Books, 1993, p. 117.

[5] Op. Cit., Fallon, p. 19.

[6] Sally Fallon, *Nourishing Traditions*, Promotion Publishing, 1995, p. 24-30.

[7] Ibid., p. 28.

[8] Ibid., p.29.

[9] *Journal of Animal Science*, 2000, 78:2849-2855.

[10] Sally Fallon and Mary E. Enig, Ph.D., *Splendor from the Grass*, www.westonaprice.org/farming/splendor.html.

[11] bid.

Chapter Summary – Recommended Actions

This chapter has presented general dietary recommendations in the form of foods that help improve digestion and achieve vibrant health. To sum it up, the following list of "dos" and "don'ts" combines information from this chapter and others, as well as some new information that will help improve digestion and elimination.

- Choose organically grown fruits and vegetables whenever possible.

- Avoid commercial meats and dairy products. Choose meat and dairy products from animals raised without the use of steroids and antibiotics.

- Avoid commercial eggs. Choose "fertile" ones, laid by "free-range" chickens.

- Add mineral-rich sea vegetables, like dulse, kelp and arame to your diet. These are good protein and mineral sources.

- Substitute unrefined for refined oils.

- Assume the squatting posture when having a bowel movement—by propping your feet on a phone book or a "Life Step™" when eliminating.

- Eliminate margarine. Substitute butter. Cook and bake with it or with coconut oil or olive oil.

- Use flax oil on foods or in blender drinks. Do not apply heat to this oil.

- Avoid refined carbohydrates—white sugar and flour products. Use whole-grains instead, and minimize their use.

- Favor the gluten-free grains: brown rice, millet, quinoa, amaranth, and buckwheat.

- Drink and cook with purified water to which minerals have been added. Do not put tap water in your body. Use a shower filter for showers and baths.

- Avoid canned and bottled juices. Make your own fresh juices—go lightly on the fruit juices; favor vegetable juices.

- Clean your fruits and vegetables (and meats too) by soaking them in a 3% hydrogen peroxide solution in a basin of water, or use a special "veggie wash" solution.

- Avoid all products containing hydrogenated oils—commercial baked goods, shortenings, margarine, peanut butter and processed cheeses.

- Read labels! Avoid or minimize use of foods with chemical additives.

- Substitute stevia or lo han for other sweeteners.

- Drink an 8-ounce glass of water with lemon juice (to taste) each morning upon rising and each evening before retiring.

8

- Drink 1/2 ounce of water for every pound of body weight daily (a 100-pound person drinks 50-ounces).

- Eliminate sodas, especially diet sodas.

- Avoid artificial sweeteners.

- Reduce intake of alcohol.

- Stop smoking.

- Reduce or eliminate coffee; use organic brews.

- Use herbal teas freely.

- Never cook in aluminum. Use cast iron, glass or stainless steel.

- Gradually increase the amount of raw foods you eat.

- Soak nuts, seeds, and grains in water overnight.

- Chew well!

- Refrigerate oils and grains—except for coconut oil.

- No deep fat frying.

- Use conventional cooking methods in preference to microwave ovens.

- Eat fruits by themselves.

- Do not combine proteins and starchy carbohydrates at the same meal.

- Use Celtic sea salt instead of table salt (available through the Grain and Salt Society—1-800-TOP-SALT)

- Avoid or limit the use of commercial dairy products. Select raw milk products if available.

- Don't boil vegetables—steam or stir-fry.

- Limit beverage consumption with meals —They dilute digestive juices.

- Do not overeat.

- Minimize consumption of high-stress proteins (pork, lamb, veal, beef, peanuts, unfermented soy, cow's milk).

- Use a fiber supplement, probiotic and an essential fatty acid supplement with lipase when cleansing.

- Use supplemental enzymes with meals— especially when cooked foods are eaten.

- Try to limit acid-forming foods to 20% of the diet.

- Breathe deeply from the diaphragm.

- Exercise regularly.

- Vacuum pack or freeze leftovers.

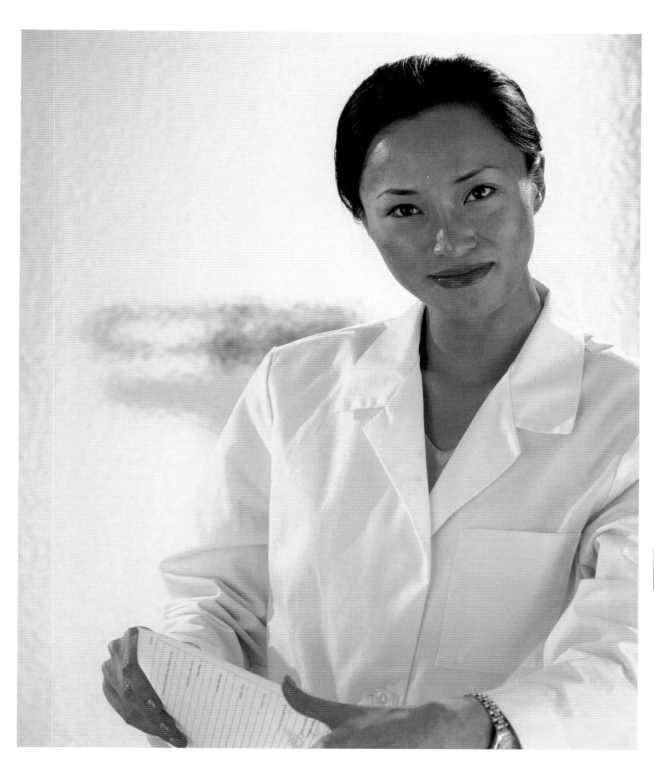

CHAPTER 9

children

In 12 children (mean age of 58 1/4 months, males) who had severe constipation of 3 or fewer stools per week, the elimination of cow's milk protein resulted in a dramatic improvement in constipation symptoms.

Source:
Clinical Pearls News, April 2002

The strongest impulse most adults feel, after their own individual survival instinct, is the impulse to help their children, to keep them safe and healthy. This is becoming an increasingly difficult task in today's toxic world where physical and mental illness are escalating rapidly.

Our children are growing up in a much more toxic environment than we did. Increases in the toxicity of food, water and air place our children at considerable physical risk. Much of today's farm produce looks good but doesn't have the nutritional value children (and adults) need. The net result of demineralization of the soil, processing of foods and widespread use of chemical fertilizers, pesticides and herbicides is devitalized, toxic food that cannot create or support good health.

To this physical stress is added the emotional stress of today's fast-paced society. Most children today are raised either in single-parent households or in two-income families. The effect is stressful for all concerned. The child in these circumstances internalizes much of that stress. Emotional stress, combined with increased environmental toxicity and inadequate nutrition, can cause a significant weakening of a child's normally strong and resilient immune system. This can result in ear or throat infections, flu and other common childhood illnesses that typically cause the worried parent and sick child to visit the doctor's office. All too often, the treatment of choice, following a cursory examination, is a broad-spectrum antibiotic. Such treatment can have the net effect of depressing immunity by killing good as well as bad bacteria in the gut, allowing for the proliferation of opportunistic infections such as candida and parasites. In this chapter, we'll look at nonmedical ways to manage these conditions in children, as well as focus on two of today's most widespread childhood disorders—earaches and Attention Deficit Disorder (ADD).

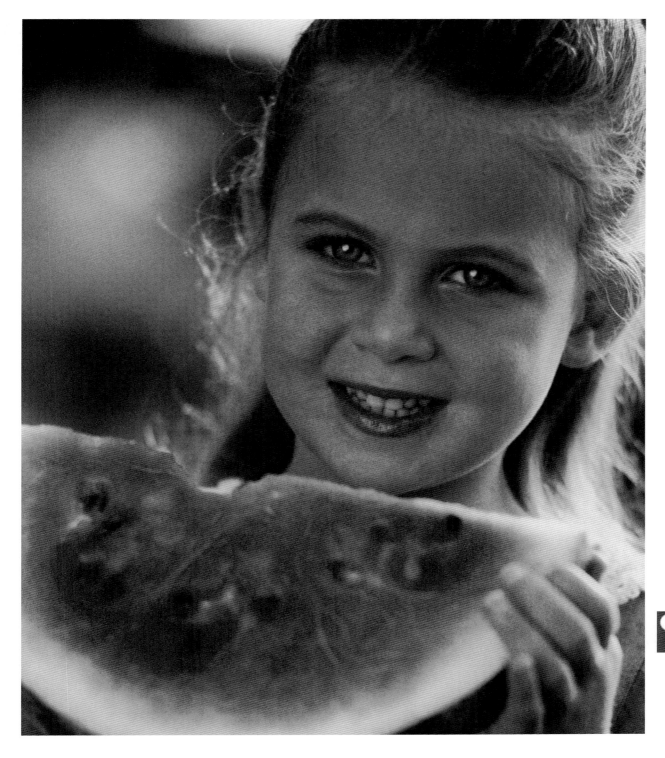

9

Earaches

An earache—technically known as **otitis media** (middle ear infection)—is *the* most common medical problem among young children today, accounting for more than 50% of all visits to pediatricians. The acute form (usually preceded by upper respiratory infection or allergy) will affect 66% of American children by age two, while the chronic form (constant swelling in the middle ear) will affect an equal number by age six.[1]

Although the standard of medical care for the condition involves use of antibiotics, analgesics (pain medication) and/or antihistamines and sometimes surgery (**myringotomy**—tubes in the ears—to drain fluid into the throat), numerous studies have shown that these methods were no more successful than a **placebo** (inactive substance) in alleviating symptoms.[2] These treatments, of course, are addressing the symptoms and not the cause and, in many instances, creating conditions for development of more serious problems.

To treat the cause, it must first be identified. As in so many other disorders, food allergies appear to have a direct relationship to ear infections. In fact, "Most studies show that 85% to 93% of children with chronic otitis media have allergies—16% to inhalants, 14% to food and 70% to both."[3] Previous chapters have noted the relationship of food allergies and sensitivities to poor digestion—how undigested proteins entering the circulation trigger an autoimmune allergic response.

Natural therapies, aimed at boosting immunity by treating food allergies, have a much better track record than drugs and surgery for treating ear infections, with "elimination of food allergens resulting in a dramatic effect in over 90% of children in some studies."[4] The same natural

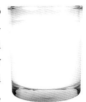

means of diagnosing and treating food and environmental allergies and sensitivities used in adults may be used for children—i.e., ELISA blood test, elimination diet and food rotation (so that no one food family is eaten too often), and desensitization techniques (such as allergy shots). In the absence of testing, one may simply remove the most common allergens (milk and dairy products, wheat, eggs, soy, corn, oranges and peanut butter) from the child's diet. This increases the opportunity for improvement. These foods may be reintroduced slowly, one at a time, after a period of several months, watching carefully for a reaction.

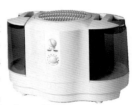

Chances of improvement are especially good if additional supportive measures are taken: Add fresh vegetable juices to the child's diet, use a humidifier if the air is dry, eliminate sugar from the child's diet (it's immunosuppressive); instead of sugar, use the South American herb stevia or the Chinese herb lo han. Additionally, supplements like thymus extract (500 mg. per day), liquid zinc sulfate (1–2 mg. four times a day) and vitamin C with bioflavonoids (50 mg. every two hours while symptoms are severe) can help enhance the immune system.

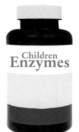

Since impaired digestion is a root cause of food allergies, it is also very important to help the child's digestion with a good plant-based enzyme taken with meals. Additionally, use of a probiotic to supplement the child's intestinal flora is recommended; this is especially important if antibiotics have been used.

It has been established that children who are breast-fed have fewer incidences of ear infection than those who are bottle-fed. Breast-feeding a baby for a minimum of four months can help prevent ear infections.[5] This may be due to the protective effect of human milk or to the elimination of the allergy risk posed by cow's milk. There is also an established connection between a child's exposure to cigarette smoke (even second-hand) and development of ear infections.[6]

Interestingly, "frequent ear infections and antibiotic use are associated with a greater likelihood of developing ADD,"[7] another common childhood disorder that is on the rise.

ADD/ADHD

The term ADD was first used in 1980. Technically, there are two types of ADD—ADD with hyperactivity and just plain ADD (without hyperactivity). Prior to 1980, children with the disorder had been referred to as hyperkinetic or hyperactive. The term "minimal brain dysfunction" was also used at one time. It reflects the erroneous belief that the condition is caused by brain damage. Usually, ADD and hyperactivity go hand in hand—making the condition ADHD (Attention Deficit Hyperactivity Disorder), though some 20% of children are diagnosed as just ADD. This condition may continue on into adulthood, at which time it's known as "ADD, residual type."

ADHD is now viewed as a psychiatric disorder char-acterized by impulsiveness, poor attention span and age-inappropriate hyperactivity. "Estimates of its incidence vary widely, ranging from 1–40% of the nation's children, with the most widely accepted range being between 3–10%."[8] Boys are three to four times more affected than girls. The disorder tends to run in families.

It has also been established that hyperactive children are more likely than those in the general population to become alcoholics, smokers and drug abusers in their adult years. ADD and addiction share distinct biochemical imbalances, which can be largely corrected through proper diet and supplementation. Both of these conditions are addressed in separate sections in *Alcohol ADDiction and Attention Deficit Disorder* (see 'books' in Resource Directory). The relationship between these disorders may be based on the effects of the drug methylphenidate so often prescribed to treat ADD and ADHD. Methylphenidate is officially classified as a Schedule II drug, meaning that its addictive potential is similar to other drugs in that class including cocaine, morphine, opium, methadone and methamphetamines. More than 2 million prescriptions for this powerful drug are now written each year, some of them for pre-school children. "Black market" sales of the drug have emerged, since crushing and snorting it can produce a high. Interestingly, the U.S. armed forces has a policy of not enlisting anyone who has been on methylphenidate. The list of side effects is astonishing. Among them are:

- Irritability
- Stunted growth
- Depression and suicidal tendencies (if abruptly discontinued)
- May lower attack threshold in the seizure-prone
- Nervousness
- Insomnia

- Skin rashes
- High fever
- Joint pain
- Headaches
- Facial tics
- Drowsiness
- Blood pressure and pulse changes
- Angina chest pain
- Cardiac arrhythmias
- Weight loss
- Reduction in white blood cell count
- Anemia
- Loss of appetite
- Hair loss
- Can cause severe reaction in combination with anticoagulant, anticonvulsant and antidepressant medications
- Internal hemorrhaging
- Abdominal pain
- Tourette's syndrome
- Memory loss
- Hostility[9]

Methylphenidate is just one of several drugs pre-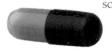scribed for ADHD children. Sadly, "there has been, every 4 to 7 years, a consistent doubling of the rate of medication treatment for such children."[10] While these drugs may be successful in controlling hyperactive behavior, too often they do so at the expense of the child's health and spirit, producing a dull, sickly, unresponsive zombie-like demeanor.

The ADD child is often diagnosed as learning disabled. Otitis media seems to factor into the learning disability portion of the ADD equation. Middle ear inflammations or infections can lead to speech impediments and delayed language development, as well as lowered IQ and learning difficulties. Ear infections are twice as common in learning disabled children as they are in other

children.[11] Prevention of ear infections therefore may also help in the prevention of ADD.

ADD may be considered another "trash basket diagnosis" when looking at the underlying factors, which may be the actual cause of the behaviors labeled ADD and ADHD. Among these are:

- Food additives
- Food allergies
- Refined sugar
- Candida and parasites
- Craniosacral dysfunction (structural misalignment of skull bones)
- Fluorescent lights
- Heavy metals

Heavy Metals

The role of heavy metals is prominent in ADD (without hyperactivity), though they may affect those with ADHD as well. This is due to a well-established link between learning disabilities (a manifestation of ADD) and a high body burden of heavy metals. High levels of mercury, cadmium, lead, copper and manganese, coupled with poor nutrition, can result in delayed development, learning disabilities and many other disorders (including criminal behavior) in children. Deficiency of virtually any nutrient can impair brain function, and multiple nutrient deficiencies are widespread among children today. Iron deficiency is the most common, and one symptom is decreased attentiveness.

All children with ADD and ADHD should be screened for heavy metals. Where found, these can be treated with chelation, a process whereby a substance is used either orally or intravenously to attract the metal and bind to it so it can be eliminated from the body. There are adult oral chelation products on the market that are natural blends of herbs, vitamins, minerals and amino acids designed to support a healthy mineral balance in the body. Though the formulas are designed for adults, they can often be used safely with chil-

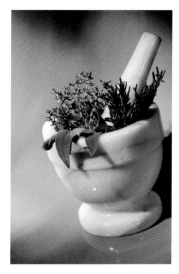

dren by just reducing the dose based on the child's weight, i.e., if the child weighs 75 pounds, and the product is based on a 150-pound person, a half dose would be given.

Heavy metals are abundant in the environment. Often they're found in the places we would least suspect, like childhood vaccines.

Vaccinations

There has been much controversy recently regarding the use of thimerosal-containing vaccines on children because of the mercury content (nearly 50%) of this preservative. **Thimerosal** is commonly used in vaccines to prevent them from spoiling; it also inactivates the bacteria that are used to formulate several vaccines and prevents bacterial contamination of the vaccine. The controversy about thimerosal reached a climax in the summer of 1999, when the American Academy of Pediatrics issued a joint statement in conjunction with the U.S. Public Health Service. It alerted physicians and the general public to the possible health threat posed by the presence of ethyl mercury (as thimerosal) in some vaccines recommended routinely for children in the U.S.

The EPA (Environmental Protection Agency) has established "safe" levels of mercury as .1 microgram per 1.0 kilogram of body weight per day. Vaccines contain 12.5 to 25.0 micrograms of mercury. Therefore, during the course of receiving a multiple vaccination during a "well baby" office visit, a child could have between 50–62.5 mcgs. of mercury injected directly into his or her bloodstream.[12]

There is a suspected link between autism (a neurological disorder characterized by impaired cognitive, social and language development) and thimerosal. Symptoms of mercury toxicity in young children are quite similar to those of autism. The increase in the number of children diagnosed as autistic seems to correlate with the introduction of hepatitis B and HIB (Haemophilus influenza, type B) vaccination of infants in the early 1990s.

Vaccinations are not the only source of mercury. It is commonly found in dental amalgam used to fill cavities in teeth. Vapors from the mercury used in dental fillings are decidedly toxic. These vapors, inhaled by a pregnant woman, can cause brain damage to the developing fetus, which can later manifest as learning disability, autism and/or ADD/ADHD. The infant who is exposed to mercury in utero via the mother's "silver" filling vapors (which are emitted every time she chews), and is then given a thimerosal-containing vaccination soon after birth, is exposed to an extraordinary amount of toxicity.

The dangers from vaccinations are not limited to the damage done by thimerosal, however. In addition to mercury, vaccines typically contain a live or killed infectious agent (usually a virus or bacteria), other preservatives (notably formaldehyde), stabilizers, antibiotics and adjuvants (such as aluminum phosphate—another toxic metal!). Hannah Allen stated that the materials from which "vaccines, serums and biologicals" are produced include such toxic components as diseased foreign tissue.[13]

9

There are many fine books on the market and sites on the World Wide Web with information on the dangers of immunizations and how to legally avoid them. We recommended the books *Immunization Theory and Reality* by Neil Z. Miller and *The Vaccine Guide: Making an Informed Choice* by Randall Neustaedter, and the websites http://think-twice. com/global.htm and www.garynull.com/market place/documents.asp.

Food Additives

The late pediatric allergist, Dr. Benjamin Feingold, was one of the first healthcare professionals to recognize a connection between food additives and ADD. In 1973, he reported to an AMA gathering that more than half of his hyperactive patients had improved on a diet devoid of artificial flavors and colors and chemical preservatives. Ironically, two commonly prescribed medications for ADHD, contain artificial color! Dr. Feingold found that many hyperactive children react to chemical compounds (salicylates and phenolics, which occur naturally in foods) and improve when foods containing these are avoided.

The U.S. uses approximately 5,000 additives in food – that's about 8–10 pounds per person per year.[14] Many of the studies that examine the effects of these additives have been funded by major food manufacturers in this country (who use them in their products). This being the case, it's understandable that Dr. Feingold's findings regarding food additives have not been consistently supported in controlled U.S. studies. It is noteworthy, however, that studies outside the U.S. *do* support the efficacy of his diet, and, most significantly, many hyperactive children have improved by following it. More information on the Feingold diet is available from the Feingold Association of the U.S. at 631-369-9340 (www.feingold.org).

While Dr. Feingold has provided a big piece of the

ADHD puzzle, a shortcoming of his diet is that it fails to address the issues of food allergy and nutrient deficiency.

Food Allergies

Studies of food allergies and sensitivities in hyperactive children have shown that artificial food colors and preservatives are among the most reactive of food substances. Eliminating them from the diet may be helpful, but frequently there are other reactive foods that must be eliminated as well. The major ones are cow's milk, soy products, chocolate, oranges, grapes, peanuts, wheat, corn, tomatoes and cane sugar.

Pediatrician, Doris Rapp, in her book *The Impossible Child*, and in the accompanying video (available through Practical Allergy Research Foundation, 1-800-787-8780), shows dramatically how hyperactivity (and other conditions) starts and stops. She uses a **provocation/neutralization** technique, wherein a small amount of the reactive food (or chemical) is introduced sublingually (under the tongue). One concentration of the allergen will trigger the maladaptive response, while another will eliminate it. In Dr. Rapp's video, children can be seen behaving normally until an allergen is introduced. Immediately, they exhibit classic ADHD behaviors and even show signs of learning disabilities. The child who wrote normally before ingesting the allergen, inverted letters afterwards. Dr. Rapp also notes that children with such food sensitivities often have distinctive physical signs: circles, bags or wrinkles under the eyes and/or a horizontal crease across the bridge of the nose.

Refined Sugar

Sugar is one of the common allergens in hyperactive children. Even in the absence of an actual allergy or sensitivity, too much sucrose causes unstable blood sugar levels, which can affect the mood and behavior.

One study found abnormal glucose tolerance curves, predominantly hypoglycemia (low blood sugar), in 74% of 261 hyperactive children.[15] Because hypoglycemia increases adrenaline secretion, it can contribute to hyperactivity. It can also lead to an overgrowth of *Candida albicans*. Where candida is a problem, sugar and other sweeteners must be temporarily eliminated from the diet. In the absence of candida, sweetening children's food with the herb lo han is recommended. It does not have the adverse effects of other sweeteners and actually helps to stabilize blood sugar levels. The same may be said of stevia, another good herbal alternative.

Candida and Parasites

Candida overgrowth is frequently the result of antibiotic overuse. Because the allergy and sugar components are so strong in ADD, the development of systemic candidiasis is not a surprising result. Recent studies and a wealth of clinical data show a close relationship between candida overgrowth and ADD or ADHD. The diagnosis of ADD or ADHD is a red flag that candida overgrowth and/or parasites may be a problem. Other red flags include:

- Thrush (oral candida)
- Colic
- Recurring ear infections
- Chronic cough
- Headache
- Constipation
- Gas & bloating
- Mood swings
- Fatigue
- Allergies
- Diaper rash
- Irritability
- Nasal congestion
- Wheezing
- Digestive problems
- Diarrhea
- Craving for sweets
- Rectal itching
- Coated tongue
- Skin problems

Dr. William Crook, well known for his book *The Yeast Connection*, has observed the presence of fungal metabolites in the urine of ADD and ADHD children. Typically, these children have a history of multiple

antibiotic use. They have been helped, Dr. Crook has found, by a sugar-free diet and antifungal medication. The same diet used for adults may be used with children. The questionnaire in the appendix of this book will help assess a child's candida risk. (Note: The adult questionnaire should not be confused with the one for children.)

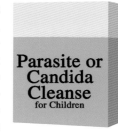

Parasite or Candida Cleanse for Children

While anti-fungal medications can help control the candida problem, it is always at a cost, because all drugs have undesirable side effects. A safer approach in treating children for candida is the use of an herbal formula. Since, as previously observed, parasites most commonly accompany candida, one would do well to address both at the same time. It is particularly important with children to treat for parasites, as children are more susceptible to them than adults for a number of reasons:

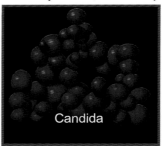

Candida

- Children have a tendency to put their hands in their mouths much more frequently than adults. The parasites on hands and under fingernails are then transported directly into the system. Playing with animals and putting hands to the mouth can be a problem.

- Children's stomachs tend to be low in HCl, which is needed to help eliminate parasites when they enter the system.

- Many children have had multiple rounds of antibiotics, which create bacterial imbalance in the digestive tract, a state ideal for parasites.

9

• Day care centers in America are rife with parasitic infection. The Center for Disease Control states that some areas of the country report as many as 50% of day care children to be infected. Parasites can be spread during diaper changing and from child to child. Additional reports state that approximately 20% of parents become infected with parasites themselves while caring for sick children.

Candida overgrowth and parasites are serious health risks for children. Clinical reports suggest that a weakened immune system and a toxic bloodstream may cause widespread systemic and nervous system disturbances. These can lead to many problems, not the least of which is a repeat of ear infections and flu-like symptoms. If these conditions are treated with antibiotics, the situation is made worse, and the child experiences a spiraling cycle of decline.

If your child suffers from frequent colds, flu, ear infections, or allergies, has been labeled ADHD or shows other signs of parasites or candida, here are some steps you can take now:

• Change the child's diet. Eliminate dairy products, sugar, wheat, corn and any products that contain preservatives or food colorings. Some good substitutes are millet, spelt, rice and quinoa. Ezekiel bread is also a tasty substitute for wheat breads.

• Vegetables are important as healing and rebuilding foods. Vegetables should be cleaned well with a vegetable wash (available from the health food store) or with diluted hydrogen peroxide.

• Start the child on a cleansing program to kill the candida and parasites from which (s)he may be suffering. A special children's formula will help to remove these pathogens. A good formula would include such ingredients as **black walnut** (aids digestion, cleanses the body of parasites), **quassia** (used in the expulsion of threadworms and stimulates production of digestive juices), **garlic** (an anti-fungal), **cloves** (has antiseptic and anti-parasitic properties), **pippli** (used in India as an anti-parasitic), **wormwood** (expels worms), **pumpkin seed** (anti-parasitic) and **thyme** (anti-fungal and anti-parasitic).

• Supplement the child's digestive process with a good **plant-based enzyme formula**, one which includes amylase, lipase, protease and cellulase and may also include **papain** (from papaya), **bromelain** (from pineapple) and **pepsin** (breaks down protein) to aid digestion, as well as **L-glutamine** and **N-acetyl-glucosamine (NAG)** and **butyric acid** to help regenerate the intestinal lining.

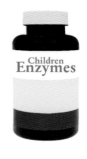

• Supplement the child's intestinal flora with a good chewable probiotic formula that includes resident strains of beneficial bacteria that will implant in the intestines. These would include *Lactobacillus acidophilus*, *Bifidobacterium bifidum* and *Bifidobacterium infantis*. A prebiotic, such as **FOS**, will help feed these flora, while added **L-glutamine** and **NAG** will help restore the integrity of the intestinal mucosa.

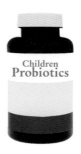

- If your child is not eliminating regularly (at least once a day), it is highly recommended that you take measures to normalize elimination naturally. A children's herbal laxative formula, containing such food concentrates as flax seed, prune fruit, fig fruit, rhubarb root and peach leaf will help in this

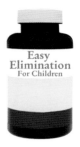

Easy Elimination For Children

regard. Herbs such as cascara sagrada or senna, which can over-stimulate the bowel, should be avoided.

Getting a child successfully through a cleansing program may require considerable patience and persistence on the part of both the child and the parents. From my experience, it is easiest to stick to a program like this when the whole family is participating. The child is much more likely to cooperate when (s)he can see the whole family is doing it. Besides—there is a strong likelihood that if a child has candida or parasites, the parents do too!

Fluorescent Lights

In the 1970s, John Ott did some pioneering research on the effects of light and other radiation on human health and behavior. His work began with plants, then animals, and moved finally to humans. In 1973, he found that when he exposed rats to the radiation from color TV sets, they became "increasingly hyperactive and aggressive within three to ten days, then progressively lethargic. By 30 days, they were so lethargic, they had to be pushed to move around the cage."[16] Such response is reminiscent of the child who is hypnotically glued to the TV set regardless of program content.

According to Ott, the same kind of radiation that comes from color TV sets also escapes from the cathodes of fluorescent lights. He also found that lead stopped these emissions of radiation. Another problem with fluorescents is that they contain an imbalance of the wavelengths that emit "white" light. Ott helped establish the fact that the human body needs exposure to **full-spectrum light** (like sunlight), which is naturally balanced in its wavelength composition.

Dr. Ott instituted lighting experiments in classrooms in a Sarasota, Florida school in the 1970s to prove his point. Two windowless classrooms were outfitted with full-spectrum lights, while two others used conventional cool white fluorescent lights. Hidden time-lapse video cameras were used to observe the children's behavior in both classrooms during a period of five months. The behavior of the children exposed to the full-spectrum lights improved significantly, as did their general attendance, learning ability and concentration,[17] while no such improvement was noted in the children exposed to fluorescent lights. Further studies have confirmed these results, and full-spectrum lights are now being used in many progressive institutions.

In view of John Ott's findings, light and radiation may be considered added stress factors that contribute to ADD/ADHD in children.

Craniosacral Dysfunction

The "craniosacral" system includes the brain and spinal cord (as well as the membranes surrounding them), cerebrospinal fluid and the bones of the skull and spine. Pioneering work in this field has been done by Dr. John Upledger who reports

9

successfully treating hyperactive children with craniosacral therapy, a system of gentle manipulation of the cranial bones to restore them to their proper positioning. He states that in his experience more than half of ADD/ADHD behavior has its roots in the craniosacral system. His institute (Upledger Institute, 561-622-4334; www.upledger.com) offers intensive programs for children with ADD and learning disabilities.

Another approach to addressing craniosacral dysfunction is a specialized cranial manipulation technique called "NeuroCranial Restructuring," developed as a refinement of an old osteopathic technique (Bilateral Nasal Specific) by Dr. Dean Howell. NCR treatment results in a widening of the skull, an improvement in the flow of cerebrospinal fluid, and thus an improvement in brain activity, according to Dr. Howell who claims that NCR creates bone changes that cannot be accomplished with craniosacral therapy. *Dynamic Healing through NeuroCranial Restructuring* (Power of One Publishing, 1-727-539-1700) has more information on this technique. ❧

Notes

[1] Michael Murray, N.D., *Encyclopedia of Natural Medicine*, Prina Publishing, 1998, p. 440.

[2] Ibid., p. 442.

[3] Ibid., p. 443-444.

[4] Ibid., p. 443.

[5] Ibid.

[6] Ibid., p. 442.

[7] Ibid., p. 273.

[8] Susan Stockton, *ADD: It Doesn't Add Up*, Power of One Publishing, 1997, p. 9.

[9] Ibid., p. 7.

[10] Ibid., p. 8.

[11] Op. Cit., Murray, p. 278-279.

[12] Alan Yurko, 'Vaccines – Injection of Death,' *Crusader*, Feb. – Mar., 2002, p. 12 – 16.

[13] Hannah Allen, *Don't Get Stuck*, Hygiene Press, 1985, p. 222.

[14] Ibid., p. 274.

[15] Ibid., p. 277.

[16] John Ott, *Health and Light*, Pocket Books, 1973, p. 127.

[17] Ibid., p. 192.

Chapter Summary

This chapter has presented information on how common childhood disorders—earache and ADD/ ADHD—can have their roots in GI dysfunction related to impaired digestion. Some of the underlying causes of these disorders—disruption of intestinal flora, food allergies, systemic candidiasis, parasites —are the same as the underlying causes in more serious "adult" diseases, like IBS.

Standard medical treatment of ear infection (antibiotics) and ADD/ADHD (Ritalin) not only fails to correct the cause of these disorders, but it also can exacerbate the conditions and/or compromise the overall health of the child with serious side effects. Conversely, safe natural approaches to healing and restoration of balance—high-fiber, non-allergenic foods, enzyme and probiotic supplements and herbal detox formulas—can be used successfully with children of all ages.

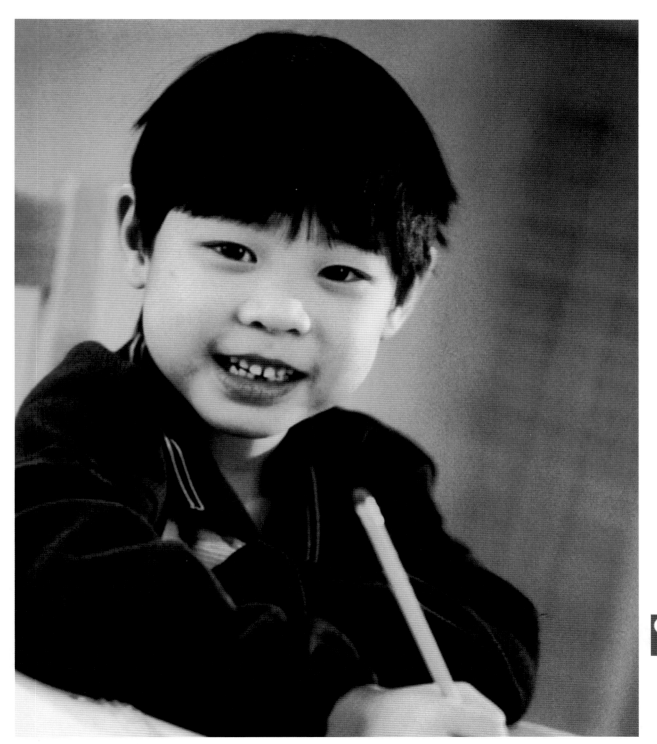

CHAPTER 10

DETOXIFICATION AND
cleansing

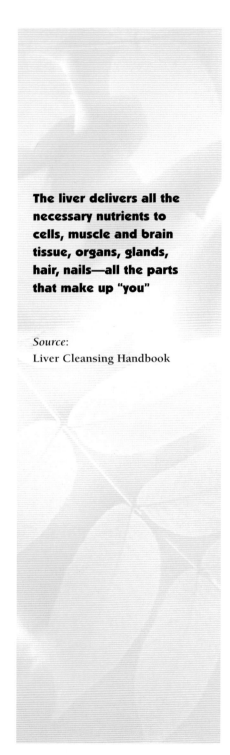

The liver delivers all the necessary nutrients to cells, muscle and brain tissue, organs, glands, hair, nails—all the parts that make up "you"

Source:
Liver Cleansing Handbook

Eliminating toxins is the third step on the road to digestive wellness and vibrant health. Cleansing and detoxification are essential to healing the digestive tract and restoring good liver function.

Detoxification is not a new concept. Many ancient cultures practiced detoxification in the form of fasting and colon cleansing with herbs. Toxins that are stored in the body can eventually overwhelm the liver. The result of this toxic overload is inflammation, which leads to chronic autoimmune disease. Toxins are foreign substances. The body will try to erect a barrier between these toxins and its own cells, organs and tissues. This barrier is inflammation, the body's attempt to protect itself from these toxic foreign substances. Inflammation can occur anywhere in the body where toxins are present. For example, if they are present in the joints, the result may be arthritis; if present in the colon, the result may be colitis. Toxic inflammation can be a direct cause of an almost endless list of chronic conditions. Even with diet improvements and a decrease in the impact of environmental toxins, the toxins that are stored in the body will remain there until removed. This is accomplished with detoxification and cleansing.

The Organs of Elimination

When asked, most people will define "cleansing" as increased bowel elimination or just colon cleansing, and they think they will have to take a laxative, stay home from work and sit by the bathroom. Because toxins are present throughout the body, detoxification and cleansing cannot be limited to just bowel cleansing. Detoxification must be viewed as a total body process for all of the body's organ systems. These organ systems are collectively called the "channels of elimination." They must all be addressed if total body detoxification is to be effective. The five (5) primary channels of elimination are:

• Colon
• Kidneys

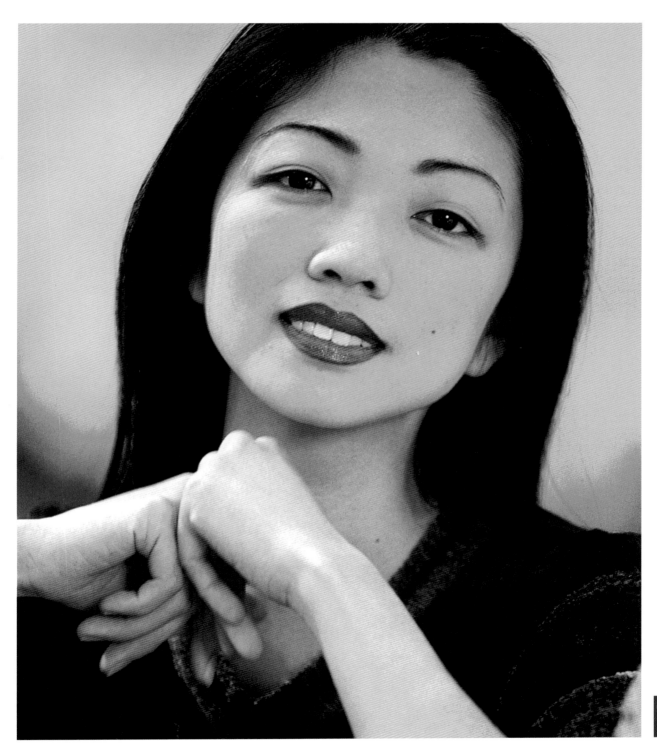

10

- Skin
- Lungs
- Liver

Colon cleansing is the very first step in the detoxification process. A clogged colon must be cleared first before embarking on any deeper cleansing programs (like candida or parasites). Most people are unaware of having a colon that is clogged and backed up with toxic waste. Unfortunately, even if people have one elimination a day, they can still have considerable waste sitting in the colon creating toxins that can eventually lead to a chronic condition. By cleansing the colon first with herbs and colon hydrotherapy, a pathway is cleared for the rest of the organs to begin to detoxify.

In addition to the colon, kidneys, skin, lungs and liver, the blood (vascular system) and lymph (lymphatic system) are critical channels of elimination that must be supported for complete detoxification to occur. There are a number of approaches that can be used to facilitate cleansing and detoxification. Some of the most effective are:

- Dietary changes
- Herbal cleansing programs
- Colon hydrotherapy
- Saunas/steam baths/skin brushing
- Fasting
- Nutrient supplementation
- Exercise

It is important to note that most of these cleansing and detoxification methods have been successfully used to achieve and maintain health for thousands of years. Exercise, rather than an energetic life-style, is a relatively recent human activity.

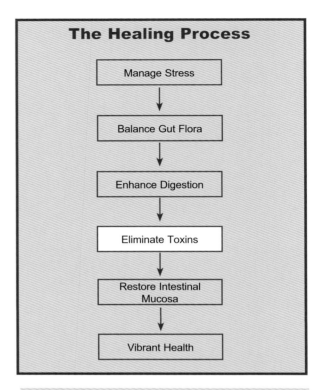

The Healing Process

Manage Stress → Balance Gut Flora → Enhance Digestion → Eliminate Toxins → Restore Intestinal Mucosa → Vibrant Health

Diet

Adhering to dietary guidelines is a very important part of detoxification. Toxins cannot be cleared while they continue to enter the body. Chapter 8 presents a good general eating plan to be followed as a lifelong prevention program.

Drinking plenty of water during a cleanse is a necessity. The kidneys cannot perform adequately without sufficient water intake. The suggested amount is 1/2 ounce of water for every pound of body weight. It is important to drink the water in small amounts (about four ounces at a time) throughout the day, rather than guzzling a large amount at one sitting, to avoid straining the kidneys. Water, means *water*, and only water—not beverages containing water (especially not coffee, tea and soda, as they often contain caffeine, which has a dehydrating effect on the body.) During a cleanse, caffeine-containing beverages should be

General Detox Guidelines
(Continue After Your Detox)

ELIMINATE	CHOOSE
• Refined sugar	• Honey, stevia or lo han
• Caffeine, soda and alcohol	• Water, herbal teas, green drinks
• Commercial salt (refined)	• Use herbs/Celtic sea salt
• Preservatives, artificial colors	• Natural whole foods
• Refined carbohydrates, white flour	• Whole grains, organic
• Pesticide-laden (commercial) foods	• Organic vegetables and fruits
• Artificial and refined oils	• Cold pressed or unrefined oils
• Processed meat	• Meat free of antibiotics, hormones and drugs
• Aspirin, Tylenol, antacids	• White willow herb, plant enzymes

eliminated. If consumed at all after a cleanse, moderation is advised.

The issue of water *quality* is as important as the issue of quantity. As previously noted, pollution is widespread today—so widespread that drinking untreated tap water can no longer be recommended. There are many types of water purification and filtration systems on the market today. The two most effective in removing pollutants are reverse osmosis (R/O) and distillation. Both methods remove all minerals along with pollutants, as there is no way to separate these. It is therefore necessary to return the minerals to R/O-treated and distilled water. This may be accomplished by using a liquid supplement that is odorless,

tasteless and colorless. Such liquid mineral supplements are available in local health food stores. Lyte Solution Concentrate, available through Health Equations (www.healtheqs.com, 1-800-328-2818), may be used for this purpose. One teaspoon of the liquid is added per gallon of purified water.

More toxins enter through the skin when bathing or showering than are ingested when drinking tap water. Therefore, some form of filtration in the shower or tub is necessary. A special zinc/copper "KDF" medium is effective for this purpose.

Herbs

The use of herbs dates to the ancient Sumerians who described their medicinal use some 5,000 years ago. The first Chinese book of herbs was written in approximately 2700 BC. Most ancient cultures relied on herbs as their only medicine. The effects of herbs on the body are well known and documented. The *Herbal PDR* (Physician's Desk Reference), the *German Monagraph E* (a resource for physicians in Germany) and the National Institute of Health's (NIH) web site, www.NIH.org, all provide extensive information on many herbs.

Even today, almost 4 billion people (two thirds of the world's population) still rely on herbs as their primary medicine.

There are thousands of herbs with medicinal properties; however, only 25 or so are used regularly for cleansing and detoxification. There are basically two types of cleansing and detoxification herbs—those used for purification and those used for revitalization. **Purification herbs** are used to purge the organ systems. **Revitalizing herbs** help soothe and strengthen the organs.

Herbal Cleansing Programs

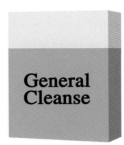

When it comes to herbal detoxification programs, you have two options: The first option is to have a customized program designed for you by a holistic physician. This might be necessary if you have moved into the "many symptoms" area of the Health Continuum (chapter 7, figure 1). The alternative to a custom program would be a pre-formulated program. This alternative would be appropriate when detoxification is part of your prevention plan (as shown on the side of the continuum towards optimal health), or when your health has moved into the "few symptoms" position.

When candida and parasites are present, it is best to start with a general cleanse before using products designed to eliminate these organisms. The reason for this is that if parasites or yeast are killed, and the colon is dirty and the liver is toxic, you may have trouble eliminating these parasites quickly enough because the colon and liver are not functioning properly.

Since most of us in today's world lead busy, stressful lives, it is of utmost importance to keep the cleansing program as simple as possible. There are two areas to address in beginning a cleanse: The first focuses on the cleansing of the colon, while the second targets the remaining channels of elimination—liver, blood, lymph, skin, kidneys and lungs—supporting them with herbs. This is *whole body detoxification*.

When the liver is overburdened with toxins, the load is passed on through blood and lymph circulation to other organs of elimination: colon, kidneys, lungs and skin. It is therefore wise to begin a general cleanse that is designed to support all of these organs simultaneously, with special emphasis on the liver. General cleanse kits are easy to use and constitute a 30-day cleansing program. Such kits should include herbs that provide support for all organs and systems of elimination. Included in an effective herbal cleansing formula would be:

Milk thistle – stimulates bile secretion, acts as an antioxidant, and strengthens the cells of the liver to protect them

Dandelion – stimulates bile and acts as a gentle laxative

Beet – helps reduce damaging fats in the liver

Artichoke leaf – stimulates secretion of bile and protects cells of the liver

Mullein, an expectorant – helps expel mucus from the lungs

Burdock – helps purge toxins that cause skin conditions

Corn silk – a diuretic to flush the kidneys

Red clover – a blood purifier and expectorant

Larch gum – helps the lymphatic system

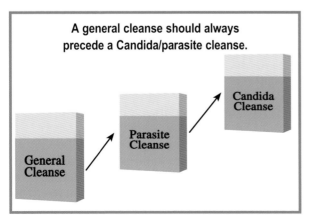

A general cleanse should always precede a Candida/parasite cleanse.

General Cleanse → Parasite Cleanse → Candida Cleanse

The formula should also include herbs to support the heart (**hawthorne berry**) and the adrenal glands (**ashwaganda**). It must also address colon detoxification. Among other colon cleansing herbs, it would contain **aloe**, **rhubarb** and **triphala** to stimulate peristalsis and **magnesium hydroxide** to regulate water in the bowel. It is very important that the colon function properly or it will not be capable of eliminating toxins from the liver. These toxins will then recirculate, creating more of a problem. Formulas like this should be taken in the evening before retiring. Kits containing these herbs that address both colon and whole body cleansing make your cleanse very easy to perform.

Fiber is also important in a preventive or beginning detox program. Cleansing stimulates the liver to release toxins into the bile, which is then secreted back into the digestive tract (via the gallbladder). It is necessary to ingest extra fiber for these toxins to be absorbed and removed in the bowel elimination. One of the best fiber supplements is **flax**, as it is a balance of soluble to insoluble fiber. **Soluble fiber** absorbs the toxins, and **insoluble fiber** sweeps the colon. Flax is also available in organic (pesticide-free) form, which is a plus. Never do a cleansing program without adding fiber for support to pick up and eliminate the toxins.

A final component in your complete body detox program would be daily intake of essential fatty acids from good quality oils. Essential fatty acids (EFAs) are fats the body cannot make from other materials and therefore must obtain from outside food sources. EFAs lubricate and soothe the colon. They are also crucial in virtually all vital functions of the body, including heart health and immunity. While there are several good sources of essential

fatty acids, some of the best are:

1. **Fish oils** – high in omega-3
2. **Flax** – high in vegetable omega-3
3. **Borage** – high in omega-6

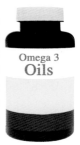

These essential oils are important in the digestive tract. A good product has the digestive enzyme lipase in the gel cap. Lipase is the enzyme that breaks down fat. It is a great way to enhance a detox program, for consuming oils without lipase puts a strain on the digestive organs.

Healing Reactions

While the net result of a cleanse will be elimination of toxins from the body, improved health and more energy, it is quite common to feel worse before feeling better. As herbal cleansing formulas kill disease-causing microorganisms such as candida and parasites, toxins are released into the system. If they are released faster than the body can eliminate them, you may experience such symptoms as fever, fatigue, diarrhea, cramps, headache, increased thirst, loss of appetite, flu-like conditions, skin eruptions or irritations. These symptoms are due to a "die-off" reaction known as the **Herxheimer Reaction** or **healing reactions**. It is sometimes difficult to distinguish between such a reaction and an actual illness. A natural health care practitioner can be of assistance in this regard. Generally speaking, the healing reaction is short-lived (a day or two, but usually no longer than a week). Symptoms may range from mild to severe, depending upon the rate of cleansing. The following steps will help to avoid, reduce or eliminate a severe healing reaction.

• Start at very low doses of your herbal cleansing formula—half the recommended dose (or less if necessary), and then gradually increase to the recommended level during a 30-day period.

10

- If liver support herbs are not present in your cleansing formula or you have a history of liver problems, support the liver with an appropriate herbal formula.
- Initiate the necessary dietary modification two weeks before starting the herbal cleanse.
- Get colon hydrotherapy sessions.
- Increase your water intake.
- Always take a fiber supplement.

A healing reaction, while uncomfortable to experience, is actually a sign of healing in progress. So, if the symptoms are mild and tolerable, there is no need to adjust the dosage of your herbal cleansing product. Try to resist the temptation to suppress symptoms with drugs: it will only increase the body's toxic load and halt the cleansing process.

Saunas/Steam Baths

The skin is our largest organ, eliminating waste via perspiration. Heat causes toxins to be released from cells into the lymphatic fluid. Since sweat is manufactured from lymphatic fluid, the toxins from the lymph are released when the body perspires. Sweating occurs naturally during strenuous activity such as exercise, exposure to the sun, or being in a warm room. Saunas (dry heat) or steam baths (wet heat) create sweat intentionally for therapeutic purposes. This "sweat (**hyperthermic**) therapy" not only releases toxins from the skin but also relaxes muscles, easing aches and pains. Releasing toxins via the skin through perspiration removes the load from the kidneys and liver, so those with impaired liver or kidney function may safely detoxify in this manner.

Raising the core temperature of the body through the hyperthermic effect has been shown to have a favorable impact upon the immune system. It is one of the few known ways to stimulate increased production of growth hormone, which helps the body shed fat, while maintaining lean muscle mass.

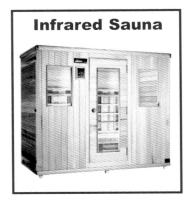

Infrared Sauna

Hyperthermic therapy also helps to restore autonomic nervous system function. This system governs muscle tension, sweating, blood pressure, digestion and balance. The autonomic nervous system is often dysfunctional in people with chronic fatigue and fibromyalgia. For this reason, people with these conditions can benefit from the two types of sauna therapies:

- Conventional sauna
- Infrared sauna

A conventional sauna heats the air either electrically or by the burning of wood. The skin perspires as a result of direct contact with the hot air. Typically, temperatures of 180 to 235 degrees Fahrenheit are used to induce sweating. These high temperatures increase cardiac load in the same way that aerobic exercise does.

Hal Huggins, D.D.S., an authority on mercury detoxification, recommends use of the sauna for detoxification. He suggests that the ill, environmentally sensitive patient start out at a temperature of 135 degrees and work up to staying in the sauna for 45 minutes without discomfort, then leave the sauna at any sign of discomfort. Once 135 degrees is comfortably tolerated for 45 minutes, temperature may be gradually increased to 145 degrees.[1] (These temperatures apply to a conventional sauna, not infrared.)

In recent years, infrared saunas have been widely used for their superior therapeutic effect. Infrared heat is radiant heat. It heats objects directly without heating the air in between. In the infrared sauna, only 20% of the infrared energy heats the air; the other 80% is directly converted to heat within the body. The result is that the body perspires more quickly at lower temperatures than in a conventional sauna. The heat also penetrates more deeply, although without the discomfort and draining effect often experienced in a conventionally heated sauna. An infrared sauna produces two to three times more sweat volume, and because of the lower temperatures used (110-130 degrees), it is considered safer for those at cardiovascular risk.

Infrared saunas have been successfully used by people suffering from sports injuries, arthritis, chronic fatigue and fibromyalgia, as well as other painful conditions. These saunas accelerate the removal of toxic metals, as well as organic toxins like PCBs and pesticide residues—chemicals that

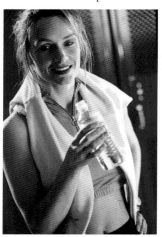

are stored in the fatty tissues of the body and are not easily dislodged. The heat produced in infrared saunas is extremely beneficial for those suffering from such skin conditions as acne, eczema, psoriasis and cellulite. The sweating caused by deep heat helps eliminate dead skin cells, and improves skin tone and elasticity. Weight loss is facilitated through use of an infrared sauna—probably due to the increase in growth hormone that it produces. It has been calculated that one can burn 600 calories in 30 minutes in an infrared sauna. Health benefits can certainly be obtained in a

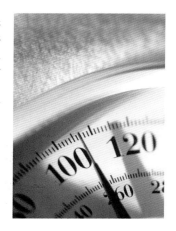

conventional sauna or steam bath as well, but the infrared sauna has a greater range of therapeutic efficiency, especially for detoxification. The infrared sauna actually has an energizing effect on users, making them feel good as toxins are eliminated.

Conventional saunas and steam baths are generally found in gymnasiums and health spas. Infrared saunas are more apt to be found in clinics run by holistic practitioners. People with health problems should consult a natural health care practitioner before using either type of sauna.

If you don't have access to a sauna or steam bath, you may want to do your own detoxification bath at home. This is prepared by filling a clean tub with hot, filtered water (a shower filter or whole house filter is recommended)—as hot as you can comfortably tolerate. There are a number of therapeutic substances that can be used in the bath water. One is epsom salts, which contain magnesium to relax muscles and sulfur to aid in detoxification and help increase blood supply to the skin. One quarter cup of salts is a good start, with a gradual increase to as much as two to four pounds per bath. Another option is ginger root. Ginger helps the body to sweat, so toxins are drawn to the skin's surface. To prepare the ginger bath, place half-inch slices of fresh ginger in boiling water; turn off the heat, and steep for 30 minutes. Remove the ginger, and pour the water into the tub.[2]

10

Dr. Hal Huggins suggests the following procedure for a detox bath:

- Bring the bath water to a temperature of 104 degrees Fahrenheit.
- Soak a bath sheet (3' x 6' towel) in the bath water.
- Get in the tub, and pull the bath sheet over you like you would a bed sheet.
- Keep the towel warm by periodically soaking it in the water.
- Leave the tub when you start to feel woozy.
- Stay in no longer than 20 minutes.
- Rinse off with fresh water.
- Repeat the procedure 2–3 times per week.

Dr. Huggins states that a soak of only two to three minutes will actually produce results, while benefits are maximized at 20 minutes. Often metals leave the body and appear after the bath in the form of a powder that adheres to the tub walls. Dr. Huggins suggests that adding a cur of baking soda to the bath water will enhance the effect of the soak. After the third bath, decrease baking soda to 1/2 cup, but also add 1/2 cup of Epsom salts. After another three baths, add 1 full cup of each.[3]

Other detox bath additives may include:

- Apple cider vinegar
- Hydrogen peroxide
- Clay
- Oatstraw (good for skin conditions)

In addition to saunas and detox baths, toxins may be eliminated from the skin by brushing it with a special natural bristle skin brush. This can be purchased in a health food store. Brush the skin before showering or bathing, stroking toward the heart, gently but vigorously. This will help stimulate lymph flow, as well as remove dead skin cells.

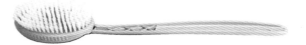

Colon Hydrotherapy

It is in the colon that the digestive process is completed, certain vitamins are synthesized, and water-soluble nutrients are absorbed. This important organ not only eliminates solid waste but also helps protect the body from infection and disease (a function of the beneficial flora). Dysbiosis can develop here, adversely affecting both elimination and overall health.

The importance of a high-fiber diet, including plenty of fruits (unless candida is an issue), vegetables and whole grains, has been explored, as has the advisability of using a balanced (soluble/insoluble) fiber supplement, especially when actively involved in a cleansing program. There is yet another way that the colon can be helped in its elimination process, and that is mechanically through the application of **colon hydrotherapy**.

Hydrotherapy is water therapy. Colon hydrotherapy then is the therapeutic application of water in the colon. The most familiar form of colon hydrotherapy is the enema. This mundane therapy has a most interesting history. Enema use dates to ancient Egypt; in fact, it is mentioned in the writings of several cultures in antiquity, including the Sumerians, Chinese, Hindus, Greeks and Romans.

Initially, enemas were a tool of the medical community, administered under the supervision of physicians. However, the practice of taking enemas (then called "**clysters**") became quite popular in the home in the 17th century. The fluid carried in the clyster was often embellished with color and fragrance, and it was not uncommon for people to have as many as three to four daily rectal infusions. Monarchs were particularly privileged in this regard: History records that Louis XIII received more than 200 enemas in one year! As time passed, "enema mania" faded, improvements were made in the process, and, by the early 19th century, colon hydrotherapy became once again the province of the medical community.

It was J.H. Kellogg, M.D., of Battle Creek, Michigan (and Corn Flakes fame), who popularized colon hydrotherapy in the U.S. He reported in 1917 in the *Journal of the American Medical Association* that he was able to successfully treat all but 20 of 40,000 gastrointestinal patients using only diet, exercise and enemas—no surgery.

Dr. Kellogg's published success with enemas led to the development of advanced colon cleansing equipment to perform the colon-cleansing procedures known as **colonics** or **colonic irrigations**. A colonic is basically an extended and more complete form of enema. Both the enema and the colonic involve the infusion of water into the rectum. However, the enema is a one-time infusion; the patient takes in as much as a quart of water, holds it for a time, and then evacuates directly into the toilet. In contrast, colonic treatment (now known as colon hydrotherapy) involves repeated infusions of filtered, warm water into the colon by a certified colon therapist, while the gowned patient lies comfortably on a treatment table.

> *Since 1976, when colon hydrotherapy equipment has been registered with the FDA, there have been over 5 million colonics administered. Additionally, in this time, there has not been one verified or validated case, or any litigation alleging injury or death as a result of the use of the colon hydrotherapy equipment from the manufacturers of colon hydrotherapy equipment that are registered with the FDA.*
>
> — In a letter from I-ACT to the California Attorney General

While water is sent through the sigmoid (only a small portion of the lower colon) with an enema, the water from a colonic travels throughout all sections of the large intestine. The colon therapist is trained to use massage techniques to relax abdominal muscles and ensure that all areas of the colon are adequately flushed. While the colon is filled and emptied a few times during one session (during a period of approximately 45 minutes), there is no need for the client to leave the table to expel the water: The passage of the water in and out of the colon is controlled by the therapist who operates the instrument. The client lies still as the water is expelled from the body. It travels through a clear viewing tube, which allows one to see what is being eliminated from the body—fecal matter, gas, mucus etc. There is no odor or health risk involved in the colonic procedure when performed properly by a trained practitioner. The therapeutic benefits of colon hydrotherapy are numerous and include:

- Improved muscle tone
- Reduced stagnation
- Reduced toxic waste absorption

10

• Thorough colon cleansing and balancing
Rheumatologist Arthur E. Brawer, M.D., lists the
following conditions among those he has found
to respond well to colon hydrotherapy[4]:

• Allergies	• Arthritis
• Asthma	• Acne
• ADD	• Body odor
• Memory lapses	• Hypertension
• Chronic fatigue	• Brittle hair
• Brittle nails	• Spastic colon
• Cold hands and feet	• Colitis
• Headaches	• Multiple sclerosis
• Constipation	• Fibromyalgia
• Irritable bowel	• Mouth sores
• Nausea	• Peripheral neuropathies
• Peptic ulcer	• Potbelly
• Poor posture	• Seizures
• Muscle pain	• Joint aches
• Chest pain	• Skin rashes
• Toxic environmental exposure	• Toxic occupational exposure
• Pigmentation	

Because of its many health benefits, colon hydrotherapy flourished in the U.S. until the mid-
1960s, at which time it began a slow decline. By
about 1972, most colonic equipment had been
removed from hospitals and nursing homes,
displaced by the use of drugs (prescriptive laxatives) and surgery (colostomy). Today, 100,000
such operations are performed annually (many
of them unsuccessfully), while 70 million
Americans who suffer from bowel problems are
spending more than $400,000,000 every year
on laxatives, according to the International
Association for Colon Hydrotherapy.

> Now, at the turn of the millennium, progressive physicians are turning once again to the use of colon hydrotherapy as an adjunct to their treatment protocols.

A number of physicians using colon hydrotherapy
(including gastroenterologists) were interviewed
by Dr. Morton Walker for the August/September
2000 edition of *Townsend Letter for Doctors and
Patients*. Their comments appear in his article
entitled "Value of Colon Hydrotherapy Verified by
Medical Professionals Prescribing It." The physicians interviewed by Dr. Walker presented case
histories and spoke of the ability of colon hydrotherapy (used alone or in conjunction with other
natural treatment modalities) to ease or resolve
symptoms in people suffering from benign pros-
tatic hyperplasia, cancer, silicone toxicity, diverticulosis, diverticulitis, yeast problems, drug and
alcohol addiction and other disorders. Dr. James
P. Carter, M.D., flatly stated that "it [colon hydro-
therapy] takes away any desire to use drugs or
imbibe in alcoholic beverages…should be part
of nearly any addict's therapeutic regimen."[5] W.
John Diamond, M.D., made the point that colon
hydrotherapy stimulates the liver, thus helping
to rid the body of debris that's sticking to the
mucosa in the bowel wall.

Many patients have been able to overcome
chronic constipation problems through colon
hydrotherapy. Unlike chemical laxatives, which
encourage dependency, colon hydrotherapy actually helps to tone the bowel, so that it resumes
normal function. Hydrotherapy sessions can
be used to "re-educate" the bowel to function
normally. The International Association for Colon
Hydrotherapy (I-ACT), headquartered in San
Antonio, TX, is the worldwide certifying body for
colon hydrotherapists. The organization works in

conjunction with local municipalities to regulate the practice by establishing training standards and guidelines. I-ACT literature describes colon hydrotherapy as follows:

...a safe, effective method of removing waste from the large intestine, without the use of drugs. By introducing pure, filtered and temperature-regulated water into the colon, human waste is softened and loosened, resulting in evacuation through natural peristalsis.

> **To find an I-ACT certified colon hydrotherapist who is using FDA registered equipment, disposable rectal nozzles (speculums) and filtered water, contact I-ACT at 210-366-2888 (www.i-act.org).**

Some people have concerns about colon hydrotherapy due to opinions expressed in articles (from some medical doctors and others) about the possibility of passing on disease and/or puncturing the colon. Such concerns are unfounded. A qualified therapist uses disposable tubes and speculums. The colonic instrument is FDA registered, so there are checks and balances to ensure its safety. As far as puncturing the colon, there is no basis for this concern. Colon hydrotherapy has been certified in the state of Florida since 1952 with no problems whatsoever. If properly performed, colon therapy is a safe, healing modality. Some people have made statements questioning the safety of colon hydrotherapy. Such statements are usually opinions expressed by people who do not have all of the information, or their documented "evidence" should be thoroughly studied.

There are two types of FDA-registered colon therapy instruments in the U.S. marketplace. These are referred to as "open" and "closed" systems. Switching from one system to another can cause some confusion for the layman.

The **closed system** is always operated by a therapist. The client is gowned and draped, and a speculum (rectal tube) is inserted in his rectum. He then turns over on his back. The therapist will fill the colon with water and empty it a number of times. The temperature of the water and the filling and emptying of the colon is always controlled by the therapist. The reason it is called a "closed" system is that the water and waste material are always enclosed in tubing and instrumentation. The waste material is disposed of through a closed drain system. The Resource Directory lists manufacturers of closed systems.

In the **open system**, the client is appropriately draped. Once the rectal tube is inserted, the therapist turns on the water. In some cases, the client may request privacy and conduct the colon therapy session himself. The open system is best described as having a single tube bringing water into the colon. The waste material flows around the tube into the base of the instrument and is expelled into the sewer. An odor exhaust system ensures the room remains odor free. The Resource Directory lists manufacturers of open systems.

A final step to improve eliminations is to simulate the natural squatting posture while sitting on the toilet. This can be done by elevating the feet, resting them on a special platform called a Life Step™.

Fasting/Juice Diets

Fasting is the abstinence from food for a period of time for therapeutic or religious purposes.

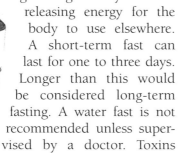

This supports the body by resting the digestive system and releasing energy for the body to use elsewhere. A short-term fast can last for one to three days. Longer than this would be considered long-term fasting. A water fast is not recommended unless supervised by a doctor. Toxins stored in the body begin to be released and could cause severe detox reactions. Also, people with blood sugar problems could be adversely affected. Most people can adequately and safely maintain a detoxification program based on juicing fresh fruits and vegetables. These supply the nutrients needed to support the body, and they require very little digestion. A juice diet is preferable to a water fast in today's toxic world.

Although it is unreasonable to eat 10 to 20 pounds of vegetables, it is easy to consume the juice from 10 to 20 pounds of vegetables during the course of a day. Even if the average person *were* able to eat that many vegetables, 90% or more of the nutrients would be eliminated in the vegetable fiber as it passes through the body. Juicing provides the full value—100%—of the nutrients since the juice, containing all the nutrients, is normally separated from the vegetable fiber by the juicer. Freshly prepared juices are quickly and easily digested and absorbed in approximately 1/2 hour.

There are many good juicers on the market today, priced from about $50 to more than $1,000. The more expensive ones are more efficient; however, even the least expensive juicer on the market will work nicely for the person new to juicing.

There are also many fine books about juicing available in most local health food stores. We recommend *Juicing for Life* by Cherie Calbom and Maureen Keane. Both of these authors have master's degrees in nutrition and provide the reader not only with tasty, easy to prepare juice recipes, but also a great deal of useful information on which juices and nutrients are most useful in treating some 50 disorders, including a number of GI problems. They recommend consuming two to four glasses of freshly prepared juice daily. "Fresh" is the key word here. As previously mentioned, juices begin to lose their nutritional value within a short time of extraction and therefore should be consumed immediately. They do not store well. The reason that juices from the supermarket stay "fresh" is that they have been pasteurized (heated in order to kill bacteria) to increase their shelf life. Usually chemical additives are used as well. There is no comparison between canned or bottled juices and freshly prepared juices. The former are nutrient-depleted and toxic to some degree because of the chemical residues they leave in the body; freshly prepared juices are rich in vitamins, minerals, enzymes and all the companion nutrients.

Step one in juicing is to buy the produce. Select organic produce, and wash it in hydrogen peroxide or a commercial veggie wash. If organic produce is unavailable, you may want to peel vegetables before running them through your juicer. The skins of most fruits and vegetables, including lemons and limes, may be left on. The skins of oranges, grapefruit, kiwis and papayas should be discarded, however. Remove pits from peaches, plums, etc., but fruits with seeds may be run through a juicer. An exception is apple seeds; these contain some cyanide so should be removed. Carrot and rhubarb greens must also be removed before juicing, as these contain toxic substances.

Any high-water-content fruit or vegetable may be used in a juicer. This would include all fruit except bananas and avocados.

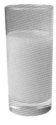

Drink four glasses (4–12 ounces each) of *fresh* juice throughout the day while on a juice diet. Also, you'll want to drink at least four 8-ounce glasses of water throughout the day.

How you end a juice diet is just as important as

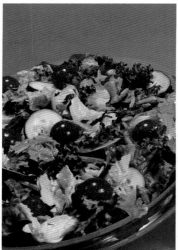

sticking to the diet. It is imperative to ease into normal eating. The first meal after a juice diet is concluded may consist of a fruit or vegetable salad with lemon juice dressing, accompanied by juice and herbal tea. The second meal could consist of the salad plus a fresh vegetable soup, plus juice. The same items could be repeated for dinner—or a steamed

vegetable may be substituted for the soup. On the second day, breakfast would be the same: juice, salad and herbal tea. Lunch might consist of juice, salad, soup and brown rice. By dinner of the second day, a potato and baked or broiled fish may be added. Ending a juice diet too quickly, with the wrong foods, can put an extra load on the body and cancel the benefits gained. This is very important to keep in mind.

Prolonged juice diets may be used therapeutically under supervision to treat serious disorders. The late Max Gerson, M.D., was noted for his success with treating cancer patients using juice therapy (13 glasses per day!) as a focal point of treatment.

A juice diet is not required to detoxify the body, and for some people, may not be feasible. Others may want to start their cleansing program with a couple of days of fresh juice; the weekend would be the best time so there is time for adequate rest. Apart from juice diets, adding fresh juice to a daily diet will support a cleansing program. The simpler the better!

Nutrient Supplementation

Those on a detoxification program can benefit from extra vitamins and minerals, particularly the antioxidants (vitamins A, C, E and the minerals selenium and zinc), as well as B vitamins. A multi-vitamin and mineral may be used to support the body as it is detoxifying toxic chemicals. Make super foods, such as green drinks, a regular part of your diet. Green food drinks provide an excellent supply of nutrients during and after a detox program. They can help to boost energy during the day. The Resource Directory includes sources for some excellent green food supplements.

> While fresh vegetable juices are highly nourishing, and a periodic juice diet can be very beneficial in ridding the body of toxins, don't substitute juice for vegetables after the diet is completed. You may certainly add juice to your diet (and are encouraged to do so), but don't exclude the veggies: The body needs the fiber provided by whole foods.

10

Exercise/Deep Breathing

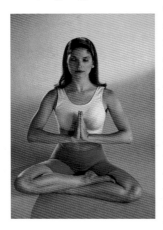

Exercise is an important element in a health-building regimen. It is also very important in the detoxification process. When we breathe in and out, the flow of lymph through the body is stimulated. It has long been known that exercise stimulates this movement of lymphatic fluid, but the role of breathing wasn't entirely recognized until technology provided the means to photograph the lymph flow process. This direct observation shows that deep breathing causes the lymph to shoot through the capillaries like a geyser. The key word here is "deep." *Deep* breathing is the kind that best stimulates lymph flow. Breathing deeply helps eliminate poisons from the cells, and also enhances immunity, since the lymphatic system is actually part of the immune system. Deep breathing enhances immunity by eliminating toxins. While the heart is the pump for the vascular system, the lymphatic system has no real pump: It depends upon movement (exercise) and breath for stimulation. Properly used, the lungs act as sort of a suction pump for the lymphatic system.

Combining deep breathing with exercise—even gentle exercise like jumping on a rebounder (mini-trampoline)—will do much to improve lymph flow and thus the body's detoxification ability and general state of health. Yoga is another tool to stimulate lymph flow, one that focuses upon stretching and controlled breathing. It's empowering to know that something as simple and (free) as breathing can be used as a powerful tool to build health.

Notes

[1] Hal Huggins, D.D.S., M.S., *Detoxification*, Peak Energy Performance, p. 19.

[2] Cheryl Townsley, *Cleaning Made Simple*, LFH Publishing, 1997, p. 47-48.

[3] Ibid., p. 23.

[4] Morton Walker, D.P.M., "Value of Colon Hydrotherapy Verified by Medical Professionals Prescribing it," *Townsend Letter for Doctors and Patients*, August/September, 2000 (#205/ 206), p. 4.

[5] Ibid., p. 6.

Chapter Summary - Recommended Actions

When you start a detox (cleansing) program, especially as a first-time cleanser, it is important to keep it simple. A realistic commitment is required to stay excited about creating long-term optimal health. Some detox options may not be available to you, or you may not be able to fit them into your schedule. The whole-body herbal cleansing program is not a one-time affair. It is best incorporated into a prevention program at least twice a year. It is the first step toward complete detoxification. Again, for people who have many health problems, it may be necessary to seek the services of a natural health care practitioner or physician who can design a custom program. Regardless of whether you choose this option or elect to use a pre-formulated cleanse, this is your first step in the detoxification process, the cornerstone of good health. Whichever option is chosen, clean the digestive system, and support the organs of elimination before moving on to more advanced cleanses, like those that address candida, parasites, heavy metals or liver detoxification. A simplified 30-day whole-body cleanse would look like this:

1. Maintain a "clean," healthy diet, one which excludes refined starches and includes the following:

    • Plenty of fresh organic fruits and vegetables

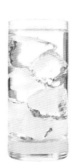

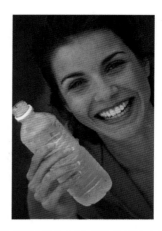

- Organic meat, used as a condiment (2 1/2-ounces per meal for women, 3 1/2–4-ounces per meal for men).
- Ezekiel bread (sprouted whole-grain)
- Herbal teas
- Purified water (with minerals added back)—7 to 10 glasses daily
- Fresh juices (optional)
- Cold-pressed (unrefined) olive oil
- Real butter

2. Take an herbal detox formula (which contains herbs discussed in this chapter) morning and night for 30 days. To help support the body in the cleansing process during this time, also add:

    a. Essential oils after breakfast and dinner (one to two capsules)
    b. A balanced flax fiber supplement before bed
    c. Vitamins, minerals after meals
    d. Super foods such as green drinks
    e. Plant enzymes (containing HCI, if necessary) with meals.

3. Skin brush.

4. Take a hot therapeutic bath, steam bath or sauna three times a week.

5. Try colon hydrotherapy at least three times or more during the 30–day detox.

6. Exercise for 30 minutes: walking, yoga or rebounder.

FACT: 75% of Americans are chronically dehydrated. (Likely applies to half the world population)

FACT: In 37% of Americans, the thirst mechanism is so weak that it is often mistaken for hunger.

FACT: Even *mild* dehydration will slow down one's metabolism as much as 3%.

FACT: One glass of water stopped midnight hunger pains for almost 100% of the dieters in a University of Washington study.

FACT: Lack of water is the #1 trigger of daytime fatigue.

FACT: Preliminary research indicates that 8–10 glasses of water a day could significantly ease back and joint pain for as much as 80% of sufferers.

FACT: A mere 2% drop in body water can trigger fuzzy short-term memory, trouble with basic math and difficulty focusing on the computer screen or on a printed page.

10

The Health Continuum

VIBRANT HEALTH

High Energy

Ideal Weight

Detoxification, Cleansing, Improved Environment

H.O.P.E. Formula, Diet and Supplements

Awareness and Education

MIDLINE

Lack of Awareness

Poor Diet

Symptoms: Headache, Heartburn, Gas

Over the Counter Medication

Prescription Drugs

Imbalanced Digestive Tract

Diabetes, Heart Disease, Arthritis, Inflammation

CHRONIC HEALTH PROBLEMS

Health is more than lack of symptoms. To maintain or regain it requires awareness, commitment, discipline and adherence to a proactive program emphasizing detoxification and rebuilding through diet and supplementation. The net result will be high levels of energy and a sense of well-being.

The road to chronic disease and disability, on the other hand, begins with lack of awareness, poor diet and symptom suppression through use of pharmaceutical drugs. Here the stage is set for the development of digestive dysfunction, which increases the body's toxic load and depletes its energy. The net result is development of more and more symptoms, leading ultimately to degenerative disease.

The Steps to Digestive Health

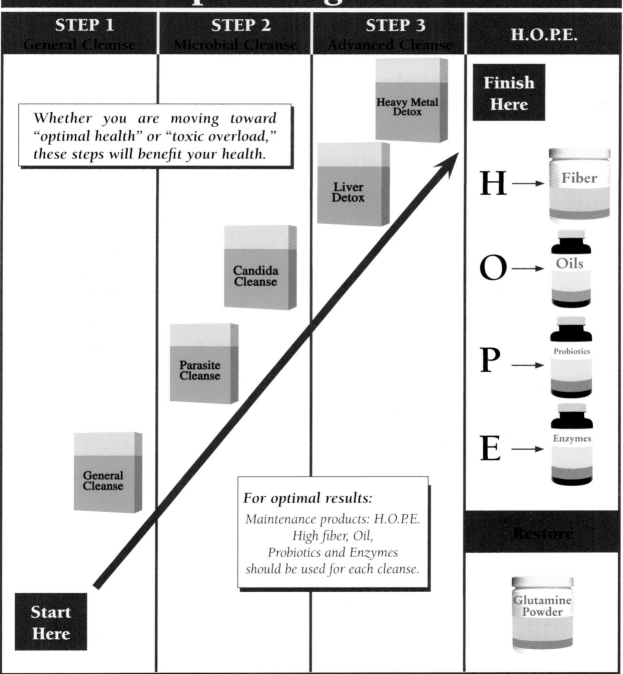

| STEP 1 General Cleanse | STEP 2 Microbial Cleanse | STEP 3 Advanced Cleanse | H.O.P.E. |

Whether you are moving toward "optimal health" or "toxic overload," these steps will benefit your health.

Heavy Metal Detox

Liver Detox

Candida Cleanse

Parasite Cleanse

General Cleanse

Finish Here

H → Fiber

O → Oils

P → Probiotics

E → Enzymes

Restore

Glutamine Powder

For optimal results:
Maintenance products: H.O.P.E. High fiber, Oil, Probiotics and Enzymes should be used for each cleanse.

Start Here

10

APPENDIX

Yeast Questionnaire – Adult

Section A – History

Circle the number next to the questions you answer "yes," then add all the circled numbers and write the total in the box at the bottom.

1. Have you taken tetracycline or other antibiotics for acne for 1 month or more? 50

2. Have you at any time in your life taken other "broad spectrum" antibiotics for respiratory, urinary or other infections for 2 months or more, or for shorter periods, 4 or more times in a 1-year span? 50

3. Have you taken a broad spectrum antibiotic drug – even for 1 period? 6

4. Have you at any time in your life been bothered by persistent prostatitis, vaginitis, or other problems affecting your reproductive organs? 25

5. Have you been pregnant...
   a) 2 or more times? 5
   b) 1 time? 3

6. Have you taken birth control pills for...
   a) more than 2 years? 15
   b) 6 months to 2 years? 8

7. Have you taken prednisone, Decadron® or other cortisone-type drugs by mouth or inhalation...
   a) for more than 2 weeks? .15
   b) for 2 weeks or less? 6

8. Does exposure to perfumes, insecticides, fabric shop odors, or other chemicals provoke...
   a) moderate to severe symptoms? 20
   b) mild symptoms?. 5

9. Are your symptoms worse on damp, muggy days or in moldy places? 20

10. If you have ever had athlete's foot, ringworm, jock itch or other chronic fungus infections of the skin or nails, have such infections been...
    a) severe or persistent? 20
    b) mild or moderate? 10

11. Do you crave sugar?. 10

12. Do you crave breads?. 10

13. Do you crave alcoholic beverages?. 10

14. Does tobacco smoke really bother you?. 10

Total Score for Section _____

Section B – Major Symptoms

For each symptom that is present, enter the appropriate number on the adjacent line:

- If a symptom is occasional or mild, **score 3 points**
- If a symptom is frequent or moderately severe, **score 6 points**
- If a symptom is severe and/or disabling, **score 9 points**

Total the scores for this section and record them in the box at the bottom of this section.

1. Fatigue or lethargy . . . . _____
2. Feeling of being "drained". . . . . _____
3. Poor memory . . . . _____
4. Feeling "spacey" or "unreal" . . . . _____
5. Inability to make decisions . . . . _____
6. Numbness, burning or tingling. . . . . _____
7. Insomnia . . . . _____
8. Muscle aches . . . . _____
9. Muscle weakness or paralysis . . . . _____
10. Pain and/or swelling in joints . . . . _____
11. Abdominal pain . . . . _____
12. Constipation. . . . . _____
13. Diarrhea . . . . _____
14. Bloating, belching or intestinal gas. . . . . _____
15. Troublesome vaginal burning, itching or discharge _____
16. Prostatitis . . . . _____
17. Impotence . . . . _____
18. Loss of sexual desire or feeling. . . . . _____
19. Endometriosis or infertility. . . . . _____
20. Cramps and/or other menstrual irregularities . . . . _____
21. Premenstrual tension . . . . _____
22. Attacks of anxiety or crying . . . . _____
23. Cold hands or feet and/or chilliness. . . . . _____
23. Shaking or irritability when hungry . . . . _____

Total Score for Section B: _____

Section C – Minor Symptoms

For each symptom that is present, enter the appropriate number on the adjacent line:

- If a symptom is occasional or mild,
  score 3 points
- If a symptom is frequent or moderately severe,
  score 6 points
- If a symptom is severe and/or disabling,
  score 9 points

Total the scores for this section, and record them in the box at the bottom of this section.

1. Drowsy . . . . ____
2. Irritable or jittery . . . . ____
3. Lack of coordination . . . . ____
4. Inability to concentrate . . . . ____
5. Frequent mood swings . . . . ____
6. Headaches . . . . ____
7. Dizzy/loss of balance . . . . ____
8. Pressure above ears...feeling of head swelling . . . . . ____
9. Tendency to bruise easily . . . . ____
10. Chronic rashes or itching . . . . ____
11. Psoriasis or recurrent hives . . . . ____
12. Indigestion or heartburn . . . . ____
13. Food sensitivity or intolerance . . . . ____
14. Mucus in stools . . . . ____
15. Rectal itching . . . . ____
16. Dry mouth or throat . . . . ____
17. Rash or blisters in mouth . . . . ____
18. Bad breath . . . . ____
19. Foot, hair or body odor not relieved by washing . . ____
20. Nasal congestion or post-nasal drip . . . . ____
21. Nasal itching . . . . ____
22. Sore throat . . . . ____
23. Laryngitis, loss of voice . . . . ____
24. Cough or recurrent bronchitis . . . . ____
25. Pain or tightness in chest . . . . ____
26. Wheezing or shortness of breath . . . . ____
27. Urinary frequency, urgency or incontinence . . . . . ____
28. Burning on urination . . . . ____
29. Spots in front of eyes or erratic vision . . . . ____
30. Burning or tearing of eyes . . . . ____
31. Recurrent infections or fluid in ears . . . . ____
32. Ear pain or deafness . . . . ____

Total Score for Section C: _____

GRAND TOTAL SCORE: _____

IF YOUR SCORE IS:	YOUR SYMPTOMS ARE:
180 (women) 140 (men)	Almost certainly yeast connected
120 (women) 90 (men)	Probably yeast connected
60 (women) 40 (men)	Possibly yeast connected
below 60 (women) below 40 (men)	Probably not yeast connected

The total score will help you and your physician decide if your health problems are yeast-connected. A comprehensive history and physical examination are also important. In addition, laboratory studies, x-rays, and other types of tests may also be appropriate.

Scores for women will be higher, as 7 items in this questionnaire apply exclusively to women, while only 2 apply exclusively to men.

If your total score for all three sections above was less than 60 for a woman or less than 40 for a man, then you are less likely to have a problem with candida. However, if you scored higher than this, then you may wish to consider lifestyle and dietary changes, as well as a detoxification and cleansing program, all of which may help you feel healthy and more energetic.

Yeast Questionnaire – Child

Circle appropriate point score for questions you answer "yes." Total your score, and record it at the end of the questionnaire.

Point Score

1.   During the two years before your child was born, were you bothered by recurrent vaginitis, menstrual irregularities, premenstrual tension, fatigue, headache, depression, digestive disorders of "feeling bad all over?"...30

2.   Was your child bothered by thrush? (Score 10 if mild, score 20 if severe or persistent)..............10/20

3.   Was your child bothered by frequent diaper rashes in infancy? (Score 10 if mild, 20 if severe or persistent) 10/20

4.   During infancy, was your child bothered by colic and irritability lasting over 3 months? (Score 10 if mild, 20 if moderate or severe) 10/20

5.   Are his/her symptoms worse on damp days or in damp or moldy places?.........................20

6.   Has your child been bothered by recurrent or persistent "athlete's foot" or chronic fungus infections of his skin or nails? 30

7.   Has your child been bothered by recurrent hives, eczema or other skin problems?.....................10

8.   Has your child received:

   (a) 4 or more courses of antibiotic drugs during the past year? Or has he received continuous "prophylactic" courses of antibiotic drugs?.................................80

   (b) 8 or more courses of "broad-spectrum" antibiotics during the past 3 years?.......................50

9.   Has your child experienced recurrent ear problems? 10

10.   Has your child had tubes inserted in his ears? 10

11.   Has your child been labeled "hyperactive?" (Score 10 if mild, 20 if moderate or severe)...............10/20

12.   Is your child bothered by learning problems (even though his early developmental history was normal)?..10

13.   Does your child have a short attention span? 10

14.   Is your child persistently irritable, unhappy and hard to please? 10

15.   Has your child been bothered by persistent or recurrent digestive problems, including constipation, diarrhea, bloating or excessive gas? (Score 10 if mild, 20 if moderate, 30 if severe) 10/20/30

16. Has he/she been bothered by persistent nasal congestion, cough and/or wheezing?. 10

17. Is your child unusually tired or unhappy or depressed? (Score 10 if mild, 20 if servere). 10/20

18. Has your child been bothered by recurrent headaches, abdominal pain or muscle aches?
    (Score 10 if mild, 20 if severe) 10/20

19. Does your child crave sweets?. 10

20. Does exposure to perfume, insecticides, gas or other chemicals provoke moderate to
    severe symptoms? 30

21. Does tobacco smoke really bother him? 20

22. Do you feel that your child isn't well, yet diagnostic tests and studies haven't revealed the cause?. 10

TOTAL SCORE: _____

Yeasts possibly play a role in causing health problems in children with
scores of 60 or more.

Yeasts probably play a role in causing health problems in children with
scores of 100 or more.

Yeasts almost certainly play a role in causing health problems in children with
scores of 140 or more.

Cultured Vegetable Recipe

Taken from *The Body Ecology Diet* by Donna Gates

Step 1 – Use mostly cabbage (organic, green and/or red), either by itself or with beets, carrots, garlic, celery, red peppers, kelp, herbs (thyme, dill), or any other vegetable you want. Use a minimum of 10 heads of cabbage.

Grind them up with a food processor. Then place them into a large stainless steel bowl, and pound them with a bat or a similar heavy, blunt object until they become a little juicy. While beating, add freshly squeezed lemon juice. (See recipe on next page).

A Champion® juicer works well for grinding vegetables, but be sure to grind them with the blank plastic piece and not the screen. This blank piece lets you grind without juicing. If you use the Champion juicer, you will not need to pound the cabbage with a bat.

Step 2 – Put the vegetables into a stainless steel, ceramic, or glass crock. Don't fill the crock to the brim because the fermenting vegetables are likely to expand and overflow.

Step 3 – Put a large portion of fresh cabbage leaves on top of the ground-up vegetables (completely covering the ground-up vegetables).

Step 4 – With your hands and a little body weight, gently, yet firmly and evenly, compress the leaves.

Step 5 – Put a plate that is as wide as possible in the crock.

Step 6 – Put some weight on the plate. You can use a jar or something else that has some weight to it. We like to use a jar that won't leak, filled with about two-thirds of a pint of water. A little weight is good, but don't put on so much that vegetable juice is forced up above the fermenting vegetables. You want to check the fermenting vegetables a few times in the next 24-36 hours to confirm you have the right amount of weight and to make sure that the plate is sitting on the vegetables evenly.

Step 7 – Cover the crock with a clean dish towel. Let the fermenting vegetables sit in a well-ventilated room at room temperature (between 60-70 degrees) for five to seven days. The longer they sit, the stronger they become. After five to seven days (6-7 days at 60 degrees and 5-6 days at 70 degrees), throw away the old cabbage leaves and moldy and discolored vegetables on the top. Put the remaining fermented vegetables in glass jars and refrigerate. This raw sauerkraut will last from four to eight months when kept at 34 degrees and opened minimally. Do not freeze.

A Beginner's Recipe
Taken from *The Body Ecology Diet* by Donna Gates

We like to add freshly squeezed lemon juice to our cabbage because it tastes delicious and retains the beautiful color in the vegetables. Here is our favorite beginner's recipe:

For every three heads of cabbage: (We use two green cabbages and one red cabbage.)

Combine 3/4 to 1 cup freshly squeezed lemon juice and 3 tablespoons dried dill weed.

Put this mixture into a stainless steel bowl, and beat it thoroughly with a blunt object. Put this into a crock or stainless steel stockpot, and cover with at least two layers of cabbage leaves, the plate and the heavy object. Find a cool spot in your house, and let it sit for six days before unveiling it. Scrape off any foam or mildew from the top or edges, and refrigerate as above. Your batch, if you've made it correctly, should be brightly colored, juicy and sweet.

If you want to add other vegetables, use a layering method:

Grate vegetables in a food processor. Add more lemon juice and more dill (or other herbs), and then pound them as explained above. Layer cabbage in the bottom of a large pot or crock about six inches deep, then add layers of carrots, peppers, beets, celery, daikon, onions, then a layer of cabbage, etc.

Press down each layer so the vegetables will be saturated in their own juice. When the container is full, cover it with the cabbage leaves, a plate, a heavy stone or weight and a dishcloth, and continue as above.

If you want to make another batch right away, some connoisseurs recommend starting your next batch of raw cultured vegetables in the same empty pot or crock without washing it each time.

You will improve your technique with each batch you make.

Resource Directory

ADD/ADHD
Feingold® Association of the United States
631-369-9340
www.feingold.org

Dr. Doris Rapp
Practical Allergy Research Foundation
P.O. Box 60
Buffalo, NY 14223
1-800-787-8780

Books

ADDiction & Attention Deficit Disorder – Suzin Stockton, Power of One Publishing (1-727-539-1700)

Beyond Amalgam: The Health Hazard Posed by Jawbone Cavitations – Suzin Stockton, Power of One Publishing (1-727-539-1700)

Candida Made Simple – Cheryl Townsley, LFH Publishing

Conquer Candida – Jack Tips, N.D., Ph.D., Apple-A-Day Press (512-328-3996)

Digestive Wellness – Elizabeth Lipski, M.S., C.C.N., Keats Publishing

Dynamic Healing through NeuroCranial Restructuring – Suzin Stockton, Power of One Publishing (1-727-539-1700)

Immunization Theory & Reality – Neil Z. Miller, Thinktwice Global Vaccine Institute (505-983-1856)

Juicing for Life – Cherie Calbhom & Maureen Keane, Avery Publishing

Nourishing Traditions – Sally Fallon, ProMotion Publishing

Root Canal Cover-Up – George Meinig, D.D.S. (available thru PPNF, 1-800-366-3748)

The Candida Albicans Yeast-Free Cookbook – Pat Connolly, PPNF (1-800-366-3748)

The Body Ecology Diet – Donna Gates, B.E.D. Publications (1-800-511-2660)

The Impossible Child – Dr. Doris Rapp, Practical Allergy Research (1-800-787-8780)

The Mysterious Cause of Illness – John Matsen, N.D., Fischer Publishing

The Pro Vita! Plan – Jack Tips, N.D., Ph.D., Apple-A-Day Press (512-328-3996)

The Terrain is Everything – Suzin Stockton, Power of One Publishing (1-727-539-1700)

The Yeast Connection – Dr. William Crook

Your Body's Many Cries for Water – F. Batmanghelidj, M.D., Global Health Solutions

Candida Information

www.yeastconnection.com

Castor Oil Pack Kit

The Heritage Store
P.O. Box 444
Virginia Beach, VA 23458-0444
1-800-862-2923
www.caycecures.com

Charcoal

New Lifestyle Health Products
30 Uchee Pines Rd, Ste. 15
Seale, AL 36875
1-800-542-5695

Clay (for Detox Baths)

LI's Magnetic Clay
1-800-257-3315
www.magneticclay.com

Chemical Sensitivities

Dr. Gloria Gilbère
Naturopathic Health and Research Center
P.O. Box 1565.
Sandpoint, ID 83864
360-352-3646
www.drgloriagilbere.com

Colon Hydrotherapy

I-ACT
P.O. Box 461285
San Antonio, TX 78246-1285
210-366-2888
www.i-act.org

Colon Hydrotherapy Manufacturers (Closed Systems)

Clearwater Colon Hydrotherapy
4451-A South Pine Ave.
Ocala, FL 34480
352-401-0303
1-888-869-6191

Dotolo Research
2875 MCI Drive
Pinellas Park, FL 33782-6105
1-800-237-8458

Prime Pacific International QPW Ltd.
P.O. Box 87076
North Vancouver, B.C., Canada V7L 4P6
1-800-223-9374

Specialty Health
21636 N. 14th Ave., Suite A1
Phoenix, AZ 85027
623-582-4950

TRANSCOM S.L.
Sangroniz, 6, Edificio Beaz
Pabellon 15
48150 Sondika (Vizcaya), Spain
001 (34-4) 4531033
001 (34-4) 4710116

Colon Hydrotherapy Manufacturers (Open Systems)

Colon Therapeutics, Inc.
2909 Main Ave.
Groves, TX 77619
409-963-0300

Tiller MIND BODY, Inc.
10911 West Ave.
San Antonio, TX 78213
210-308-8888
800-939-1110

Craniosacral Therapy

The Upledger Institute, Inc.®
11211 Prosperity Farms Rd., Ste. D-325
Palm Beach Gardens, FL 33410
561-622-4334
www.upledger.com

Dental Information (Holistic) and Referral

DAMS (Dental Amalgam Mercury Syndrome)
1-800-311-6265
www.dams.cc

Electrolytes

Health Equations
P.O. Box 323
Newfane, VT 05345
1-800-328-2818
www.healtheqs.com

Environmental Products

Healthy Home Center
2435 9th St. North
St. Petersburg, FL 33704
1-800-583-9523
www.healthyhome.com

Food Safety

Food and Water, Inc.
P.O. Box 543
Montpelier, VT 05601
fax 802-229-6751
1-800-EAT-SAFE
www.foodandwater.org

Green Drinks

Greens Plus®
Orange Peel Enterprises
2183 Ponce de Leon Circle
Vero Beach, FL 32960
1-800-643-1210
www.greensplus.com

Perfect Food™
Garden of Life
1449 Jupiter Park Drive, Ste. 16
Jupiter, FL 33458
1-800-622-8986
fax 561-575-5488
www.gardenoflifeusa.com

Sweet Wheat, Inc.
P.O. Box 187
Clearwater, FL 33757
1-888-227-9338
fax 727-462-5454
www.sweetwheat.com

Herbal Cleansing Products

Renew Life Formulas, Inc.
2076 Sunnydale Blvd.
Clearwater, FL 33765
1-800-830-4778
www.renewlife.com

Hemorrhoids

Pilex®
25675 Meadowview Ct.
Salinas, CA 93908-9396
831-484-7820
1-800-745-3995 (10-8 EST)
fax: 831-484-2203
www.varicose.com

Kefir

Helios Nutrition Limited
318 The Decotah Building
370 Selby Ave.
St. Paul, MN 55102
651-298-8565
fax 651-298-0602

Laboratory Testing

Doctor's Data™ (nutritional, gastrointestinal, immunology, environmental testing)
3755 Illinois Ave.
St. Charles, IL 60174-2420
1-800-323-2784
www.doctorsdata.com

Great Smokies Diagnostic Laboratory/Genovations™
(endocrinology, gastrointestinal, immunology,
nutritional, metabolic testing)
63 Zillicoa St.
Asheville, NC 28801
1-800-522-4762
fax 1-828-252-9303
www.gsdl.com

NeuroCranial Restructuring

NeuroCranial Restructuring
Dr. Dean Howell
2840 Northup Way, Ste. 104
Bellevue, WA 98004
1-888-252-0411
fax 888-252-0411
www.drdeanhowell.com

Nutrition

Price-Pottenger Nutrition Foundation
7890 Broadway
Lemon Grove, CA 91945
1-800-366-3748
fax 619-433-3136
www.price-pottenger.org

The Weston A. Price Foundation
4200 Wisconsin Ave., N.W.
Washington, DC 20007
202-333-HEAL
www.westonaprice.org

Sauna (Infrared)

TheraSauna™
1021 State St.
Bettendorf, IA 52722
1-888-729-7727
www.therasauna.com

Vaccinations

Thinktwice Global Vaccine Institute
P.O. Box 9638
Santa Fe, NM 87504
505-983-1856
Http://thinktwice.com/global.htm

Vacuum Packaging Systems

Tilia, Inc.™
P.O. Box 194530
San Francisco, CA 94119-4530
1-877-804-5383
www.foodsaver.com

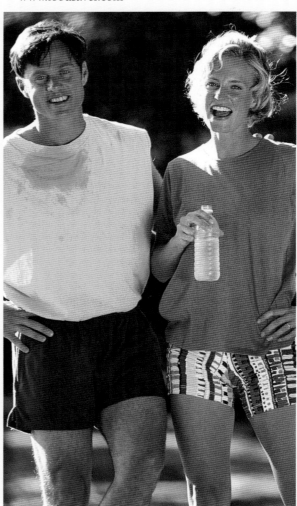

Bibliography

Batmanghelidj, F., M.D. *Your Body's Many Cries for Water*. Global Health Solutions: Falls Church, VA, 1992.

Bieler, Henry F., M.D. *Food is Your Best Medicine*. Ballantine Books: New York, 1965.

Bland, Jeffrey, Ph.D. *The 20-Day Rejuvenation Diet Program*. Keats Publishing, Inc.: New Canaan, Connecticut, 1997.

Braly, James, M.D., and Laura Torbet. *Dr. Braly's Food Allergy and Nutrition Revolution*. Keat's Publishing, Inc.: New Canaan, Connecticut, 1992.

Calbhom, Cherie and Maureen Keane, *Juicing for Life*. Avery, 1992.

Connolly, Pat. *The Candida Albicans Yeast-Free Cookbook*, 2nd Edition. Keats Publishing: Los Angeles, CA, 2000.

Erasmus, Udo. *Fats that Heal, Fats that Kill*. Alive Books: Burnaby BC Canada, 1993.

Fallon, Sally, *Nourishing Traditions*. Promotion Publishing: San Diego, CA, 1995.

Galland, Leo, MD. *The Four Pillars of Healing*. Random House: New York, 1997.

Gates, Donna. *The Body Ecology Diet*. B.E.D. Publications: Atlanta, GA, 1996.

Ghen, Mitchell J. *The Advanced Guide to Longevity Medicine*. Partners in Wellness: Landrum, SC, 2001.

Howell, Dr. Edward. *Enzyme Nutrition*. Avery Publishing Group, Inc.: Wayne, New Jersey, 1985.

Huggins, Hal, D.D.S., M.S. *Detoxification*. Peak Energy Performance: Colorado Springs, CO.

Kaufmann, Doug A. *The Fungus Link*. MediaTrition: Rockwell, TX, 2000.

Kitchen, Judy, "Hypochlorhydria: A Review – Part I," *The Townsend Letter for Doctors and Patients*. October, 2001.

Kellas, William R., Ph.D and Andrea Sharon Dworkin, N.D. *Surviving the Toxic Crisis*. Professional Preference: Olivenhain, CA, 1996.

Krohn, Jacqueline, M.D., and Frances Taylor, M.A. *Natural Detoxification*. Hartley and Marks Publishers, Inc.: Vancouver, BC, Canada, 2000.

Lake, Rhody. *Liver Cleansing Handbook*. Alive Books: Vancouver, Canada, 2000.

Lipski, Elizabeth, M.S., C.C.N. *Digestive Wellness*. Keats Publishing, Inc.: New Canaan, Connecticut, 1996.

Lorenzani, Shirley S., Ph.D. Candida: *A Twentieth Century Disease*. Keats Publishing: New Canaan, CT, 1986.

Matsen, Jonn, N.D. *The Mysterious Cause of Illness*. Fischer Publishing Corporation: Canfield, Ohio, 1987.

Meinig, George E., D.D.S, F.A.C.D. *Root Canal Cover Up*. Bion Publishing: Ojai, CA, 1993.

Murray, Michael, N.D., and Joseph Pizzorno, N.D. *Encyclopedia of Natural Medicine*. Prima Publishing, 1998.

Nichols, Trent W., M.D., and Nancy Faass, M.S.W., M.P.H. *Optimal Digestion*. Quill, An Imprint of Harper Collins Publishers, 2000.

Ott, John. *Health and Light*. Pocket Books: New York, New York, 1973.

Palmer, Melissa, M.D. *Hepatitis and Liver Disease*. Avery Publishing Group: Garden City Park, New York, 2000.

Reams, Carey A. *Choose Life or Death*. Holistic Laboratories, Inc.: Tampa, FL., 1990.

Rockwell, Sally J., Ph.D. *Coping with Candida Cookbook*: Seattle, Washington, 1996.

Stockton, Suzin. *ADD: It Doesn't Add Up!* Power of One Publishing: Clearwater, FL, 1997.

Stockton, Suzin. *Beyond Amalgam: The Health Hazard Posed by Jawbone Cavitations*, Third Printing. Power of One Publishing: Clearwater, FL, 2001.

Stockton, Suzin. *Dynamic Healing through NeuroCranial Restructuring*. Power of One Publishing: Clearwater, FL, 1999.

Stockton, Suzin. *The Terrain is Everything*. Power of One Publishing: Clearwater, FL, 2000.

Tips, Jack, N.D., Ph.D. *Conquer Candida*. Apple-A-Day Press: Austin, TX, 1995.

Tips, Jack, N.D., Ph.D. *The Pro Vita! Plan*. Apple-A-Day Press: Austin, TX, 1999.

Tips, Jack, N.D., Ph.D. *Your Liver…Your Lifeline*. Apple-A-Day Press: Austin, TX, 1993.

Townsley, Cheryl. *Candida Made Simple*. LFH Publishing: Littleton, CO, 1999.

Townsley, Cheryl. *Cleansing Made Simple*. LFH Publishing: Littleton, CO, 2001 (revised edition).

Walker, Morton, D.P.M. "Value of Colon Hydrotherapy Verified by Medical Professionals Prescribing It." *Townsend Letter for Doctors and Patients*. August/September, 2000 (#205/206).

Webster, David. *Achieving Maximum Health*. Hygeia Publishing: Cardiff, CA, 1995.

Wilson, Denis, M.S. *Doctor's Manual for Wilson's Syndrome*, 3rd Edition. Muskeegee Medical Publishing Company: USA, 1991.

Acknowledgment
Technical illustrations provided by
Dorling Kindersley© London, England

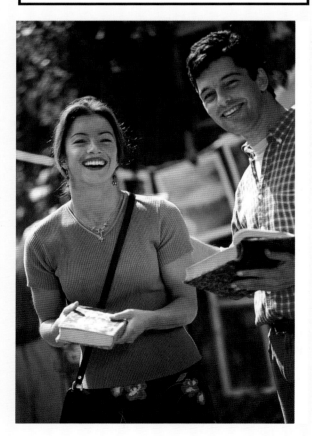

Notes:

Notes:

Notes: